A D

nutrition
assessment

SECOND EDITION

PAMELA CHARNEY, PhD, RD

AINSLEY M. MALONE, MS, RD, CNSD

American Dietetic Association
Chicago, Illinois

Diana Faulhaber, Publisher
Elizabeth Nishiura, Production Manager

American Dietetic Association
120 South Riverside Plaza, Suite 2000
Chicago, IL 60606
www.eatright.org

The views expressed in this publication are those of the authors and do not necessarily reflect policies and/or official positions of the American Dietetic Association. Mention of product names in this publication does not constitute endorsement by the authors or the American Dietetic Association. The American Dietetic Association disclaims responsibility for the application of the information contained herein.

10 9 8 7 6 5 4 3 2 1

Library of Congress Cataloging-in-Publication Data

ADA pocket guide to nutrition assessment / [edited by] Pamela Charney, Ainsley M. Malone. — 2nd ed.
    p. ; cm.
  Includes bibliographical references and index.
  ISBN 978-0-88091-421-5
  1. Nutrition—Evaluation—Handbooks, manuals, etc.   I. Charney, Pamela, 1958– II. Malone, Ainsley.   III. American Dietetic Association. IV. Title: Pocket guide to nutrition assessment.   V. Title: Nutrition assessment.
  [DNLM: 1. Nutrition Assessment—Handbooks.   2. Nutritional Requirements—Handbooks.   3. Nutritional Status—Handbooks. 4. Physical Examination—methods—Handbooks. QU 39 A1912 2009]

  RC621.A32 2009
  616.3'9075—dc22

                                         2008020723

contents

contributors

Pamela Charney, PhD, RD
Clinical Coordinator
Graduate Coordinated Program in Dietetics
Lecturer, Department of Epidemiology
Nutrition Sciences Program
School of Public Health and Community Medicine
and
Affiliate Associate Professor
School of Pharmacy
University of Washington
Seattle, WA

Gail Cresci, MS, RD, CNSD
Assistant Professor of Surgery
Director Surgical Nutrition Services
Medical College of Georgia
Augusta, GA

M. Patricia Fuhrman, MS, RD, FADA, CNSD
Nutrition Specialist
DCRX Infusion
Ballwin, MO

Jennifer Lefton, MS, RD, CNSD
Clinical Dietitian
Washington Hospital Center
Washington, DC

Ainsley M. Malone, MS, RD, CNSD
Nutrition Support Team
Pharmacy Department
Mt. Carmel West Hospital
Columbus, OH

Mary Marian, MS, RD, CSO
Clinical Nutrition Specialist, Curriculum Coordinator,
and Adjunct Lecturer
University of Arizona—College of Medicine &
Nutritional Sciences
Tucson, AZ

Mary Russell, MS, RD, CNSD
Director, Nutrition Services
University of Chicago Medical Center
Chicago IL

Cheryl W. Thompson, PhD, RD, CNSD
Vice President for Health Promotion and Education
MD Informatics, LLC
Salt Lake City, UT

reviewers

Patricia S. Anthony, MS, RD
Nestlé Nutrition—Healthcare Nutrition
Gland, Switzerland

Sara A. Blackburn, RD, DSc
Indiana University School of Health
& Rehabilitation Sciences
Indianapolis, IN

David Frankenfield, MS, RD, CNSD
Milton S. Hershey Medical Center
Hershey, PA

Jennifer A. Wooley, MS, RD, CNSD
The University of Michigan Hospitals
and Health Centers
Ann Arbor, MI

acknowledgments

Five years ago as the finishing touches were being made to the first edition of the *ADA Pocket Guide to Nutrition Assessment*, we were looking forward to its release and being able to provide a readily available pocket guide incorporating a wide variety of assessment tools and information. We never anticipated the positive response to the *Pocket Guide* and are tremendously thankful to all of you who chose to use this in your practice. Your suggestions and comments about how we could make the book an even better reference have been incorporated into this edition. We thank you for your insight and hope you find this edition just as valuable.

A significant number of dedicated individuals have been instrumental in the creation of the *ADA Pocket Guide to Nutrition Assessment,* Second Edition. We would like to gratefully acknowledge all who have shared in its creation. We cannot provide adequate thanks and appreciation to our remarkable authors. Their commitment, expertise, and patience have resulted in an outstanding resource that will assist many clinicians in their practice. We also thankfully acknowledge our reviewers who provided constructive comments and offered many suggestions to make this edition a highly useful resource.

As with the previous pocket guides, we encountered many technical issues particular to the production of this style of publication. We wish to thank Diana Faulhaber, Publisher at the American Dietetic Association, along with Pamela Woolf, Development Editor, for their ongoing guidance and support. We also wish to thank Elizabeth

Nishiura, Production Manager, for her tireless assistance in many components during the production phase.

And lastly, and of greatest importance, we would like to express our deepest gratitude to our families for their ongoing support and guidance throughout the entire creation and production of this publication.

PAMELA CHARNEY PHD, RD
AINSLEY M. MALONE MS, RD, CNSD

what's new
in the second edition
of the *ADA Pocket Guide to*
Nutrition Assessment

The Nutrition Care Process (NCP) was approved by the House of Delegates of the American Dietetic Association shortly after the first edition of the *ADA Pocket Guide to Nutrition Assessment* was published. Therefore, in this edition, we've focused on ensuring that each chapter describes fully the aspects of nutrition assessment, the first step of the NCP. Also, we have incorporated input from students, interns, and clinicians regarding changes we could make to improve readability, include new information, and remove sections that just didn't work out well.

Each chapter has been revised to ensure that we fully described each of the components of nutrition assessment. These components include patient/client history; nutrition-focused physical examination findings; biochemical data, medical tests, and procedures; anthropometric measurements; and food/nutrition history. Each component is fully described in its own chapter. Clinicians using this edition of the *ADA Pocket Guide to Nutrition Assessment* can be assured that information is consistent with the NCP.

Chapter 1 includes descriptions of two new brief nutrition screening tools along with an updated description of the differences between nutrition screening and nutrition assessment. The latest updates from the Joint Commission regarding nutrition screening are also included. Clinicians and managers alike will gain valuable insight into the screening and assessment processes as well as examples of how to do them right.

Chapter 2 has vital information for the clinician seeking a ready resource about drug-nutrient interactions. We worked to make this information as user-friendly as possible by listing drugs that commonly require patient education on potential interactions and by identifying interactions associated with different medication types. Chapter 2 also includes handy references for patient/client history information needed for different patient populations across the life cycle.

In Chapter 3, we've reformatted tables so clinicians learning how to do a nutrition-focused physical assessment can quickly find information. Chapter 4 has expanded information on gestational diabetes, completely revised tables, and new information on extracellular fluid volume.

Readers of the first edition of the *ADA Pocket Guide to Nutrition Assessment* told us they wanted a quicker way to find information on methods to measure anthropometrics and interpret the information gathered. We revised Chapter 5 to make examples of each equation easier to find and interpret. Interpretation of body mass index (BMI) in different populations and a section on measurement and interpretation of waist circumference are also new to the Second Edition.

Chapter 6 has a brand new discussion of the American Dietetic Association Evidence Analysis Library recommendations for determining energy requirements for acutely and critically ill patients. We also included several equations commonly used in clinical practice with instructions for use. All tables and information, including the highly useful electrolyte repletion protocols, were reviewed and revised to ensure that we provide you with the most current information regarding patients' nutrient requirements.

In response to questions regarding the Nutrition Care Process and how it applies in practice, we included a brand new chapter on the NCP (Chapter 7). We show readers how data from the nutrition assessment step of the NCP lead the clinician to identification of the correct nutrition diagnosis. Because the NCP and the Standards of Practice/ Standards of Professional Performance for Registered Dietitians advocate that RDs use critical thinking, we provide in Chapter 7 some new information about the diagnostic thought process. Here, we give the clinician a straightforward explanation of the components of the NCP along with a description of how health care clinicians identify a diagnosis. This is must-read information for RDs wanting to fully implement the NCP in practice!

We are confident you will find this newest edition to the *ADA Pocket Guide to Nutrition Assessment* a valuable resource for your practice. We welcome and encourage your thoughts and comments for future editions.

foreword

Nutrition assessment is an essential component of the care and management of patients in all health care settings and community programs. Assessment is the first step of the Nutrition Care Process and provides the foundation for the nutrition diagnosis. A number of basic and advanced practice skills are required to perform a complete and accurate nutrition assessment, but critical thinking is a key element required by the registered dietitian (RD). Knowledge, skills, evidence-based decision-making, and professionalism are necessary for reliable performance.

Pamela Charney, Ainsley Malone, and the chapter contributors share their valuable expertise and clinical experience in the second edition of the *ADA Pocket Guide to Nutrition Assessment*. The revised *Pocket Guide* provides up-to-date and state-of-the-art information on the tools and techniques of nutrition assessment. New to this edition of the *Pocket Guide* are data from the American Dietetic Association Evidence Analysis Library about the use of predictive equations and the determination of energy requirements as well as a chapter about how to implement the Nutrition Care Process. Samples of assessment tools and forms used in many different practice settings provide models for institutions to adopt or adapt. Charts and graphic presentations offer quick reference tools that practitioners can use to assess nutrition and hydration status, body composition, and nutrient deficiencies or excesses. Beginning with screening and progressing through history taking, conducting the physical assessment, laboratory assessment, anthropometrics, and determining nutrient requirements, the text emphasizes interpretation and application of the findings for individual patients.

Nutrition assessment by RDs has progressed from a passive activity of medical record review and patient observation for signs and symptoms of nutrient deficiency or excess to an active process of hands-on physical assessment. The authors not only comprehensively describe nutrition assessment techniques but also carefully guide the RD in organizing and evaluating data to make professional judgments and decisions. RDs are challenged to expand skills but also to engage in dialogue and discussion and critical thinking by linking practice, education, and research. My *Pocket Guide,* with all of its wonderful "tools of the trade," goes with me on patient rounds, to the office, and on home visits. The *ADA Pocket Guide to Nutrition Assessment,* Second Edition, belongs in the lab coat or on the desk of every registered dietitian!

MARION F. WINKLER, PHD, RD
Senior Clinical Teaching Associate of Surgery
Alpert Medical School of Brown University
and
Surgical Nutrition Specialist
Rhode Island Hospital
Providence, Rhode Island

chapter 1

Nutrition Screening and Nutrition Assessment

Pamela Charney, PhD, RD,
and Mary Marian, MS, RD, CSO

Despite significant advancements made in medical care, the prevalence of malnutrition in hospitalized patients remains high, reportedly ranging from 30% to 50%, with a larger number at risk for becoming malnourished (1–3). It is generally agreed that a percentage of patients in acute, chronic, and alternate-site care settings may have more complications due to their poor nutritional state (1,2). These complications may lead to increased morbidity, mortality, length of stay, and cost of care (4,5). Timely, appropriate nutrition intervention may result in improved outcomes in many care settings (6–10). Therefore, nutrition screening, the entry to the Nutrition Care Process (NCP), ensures that patients or clients in a variety of health care settings receive appropriate and timely medical nutrition therapy and is a critical component of quality nutrition care (11).

SCREENING

Overview

Nutrition screening is defined as "the process of identifying characteristics known to be associated with nutrition problems with the purpose of identifying individuals who are malnourished or at nutritional risk" (11,12). All populations, regardless of setting (acute care, subacute care, long-term care, outpatient, or home) or age, should be screened to determine the need for nutrition assessment. Screening is considered a supportive system to the Nutrition Care Process and Model (NCPM) because the screen can be conducted by individuals other than the registered dietitian (RD) (11).

The importance of nutrition screening in the health care arena has been recognized. Patients in both acute and long-term care are at the highest risk of developing nutrient deficiencies and nutrition-related complications (13). Because nutrient deficiencies or excesses often exist *before* admission (14) and may not be readily apparent (15), screening for nutritional risk in outpatient settings—including the emergency room, ambulatory clinics, and home care—is important.

Each facility or setting is responsible for determining the most appropriate mechanism for screening patients or clients. There are very few screens that have been validated (16,17). It is important to evaluate parameters used for screening to determine whether the screen is indeed identifying at-risk patients (Box 1.1).

Box 1.1 Criteria Often Used for Nutrition Screening

• Height	• Change in appetite
• Weight	• Nausea/vomiting
• Unintentional change in weight	• Bowel habits
• Food allergies	• Chewing/swallowing ability
• Diet	• Diagnosis
• Laboratory data: albumin, hematocrit (only if laboratory turnaround time is rapid)	

An effective screening process, which can be completed by any qualified health care professional, is:

- Simple
- Efficient
- Quick
- Reliable
- Inexpensive
- Low risk to the individual being screened, and
- Has acceptable levels of sensitivity, specificity, and positive and negative predictive values

Of the parameters listed in Box 1.1, only unintentional weight change and decreased appetite/intake have been validated as indicators of nutritional status (16,17). The use of laboratory values as a measure of nutritional status should be carefully scrutinized, as levels of serum hepatic proteins are indicators of severity of illness and do not reflect nutritional status. Performance of nutritional risk screening programs should be monitored and evaluated at regular intervals in order to determine whether the screen is accurately identifying those patients who require nutrition assessment and intervention. Protocols should be established in all health care settings to create a time frame for rescreening of those patients who did not require nutrition assessment at admission but have an extended length of stay. An intervention strategy should also be in place to ensure consistent and accurate communication of the results of the nutritional risk screen to the RD.

Guidelines and Sample Screens

The algorithm in Figure 1.1 (18) was developed by the American Society for Parenteral and Enteral Nutrition (ASPEN) to provide guidelines for adult nutrition screening and assessment.

Figure 1.1 Adult Nutrition Screening and Assessment Alogrithm

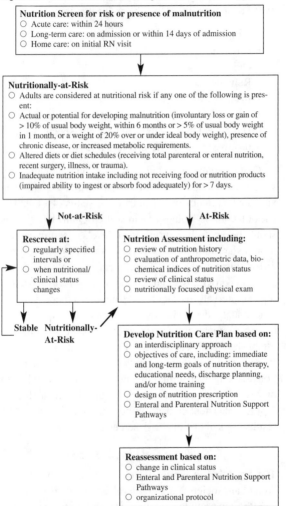

Nutrition Screen for risk or presence of malnutrition
- ○ Acute care: within 24 hours
- ○ Long-term care: on admission or within 14 days of admission
- ○ Home care: on initial RN visit

Nutritionally-at-Risk
- ○ Adults are considered at nutritional risk if any one of the following is present:
- ○ Actual or potential for developing malnutrition (involuntary loss or gain of > 10% of usual body weight, within 6 months or > 5% of usual body weight in 1 month, or a weight of 20% over or under ideal body weight), presence of chronic disease, or increased metabolic requirements.
- ○ Altered diets or diet schedules (receiving total parenteral or enteral nutrition, recent surgery, illness, or trauma).
- ○ Inadequate nutrition intake including not receiving food or nutrition products (impaired ability to ingest or absorb food adequately) for > 7 days.

Not-at-Risk

At-Risk

Rescreen at:
- ○ regularly specified intervals or
- ○ when nutritional/ clinical status changes

Nutrition Assessment including:
- ○ review of nutrition history
- ○ evaluation of anthropometric data, biochemical indices of nutrition status
- ○ review of clinical status
- ○ nutritionally focused physical exam

Stable Nutritionally-At-Risk

Develop Nutrition Care Plan based on:
- ○ an interdisciplinary approach
- ○ objectives of care, including: immediate and long-term goals of nutrition therapy, educational needs, discharge planning, and/or home training
- ○ design of nutrition prescription
- ○ Enteral and Parenteral Nutrition Support Pathways

Reassessment based on:
- ○ change in clinical status
- ○ Enteral and Parenteral Nutrition Support Pathways
- ○ organizational protocol

Table 1.1 (16) is an example of a rapid screen that can be completed, by nursing or other ancillary personnel, when a patient is admitted to the hospital. This tool has been found to be valid and reliable in identifying patients in acute-care settings who require nutrition assessment.

Table 1.1   Rapid Nutrition Screen for Hospitalized Patients (Malnutrition Screening Tool)

Parameter	Score
Have you lost weight recently without trying?	
No	0
Unsure	2
If yes, how much weight (kilograms) have you lost?	
1–5	1
6–10	2
11–15	3
> 15	4
Unsure	2
Have you been eating poorly because of a decreased appetite?	
No	0
Yes	1
Total	

Score of 2 or more = patient at risk for malnutrition.

Reprinted with permission from Ferguson M, Capra S, Bauer J, Banks M. Development of a valid and reliable malnutrition screening tool for adult acute hospital patients. *Nutrition.* 1999;15:458–464.

Table 1.2 (19) is an example of another simple nutrition screening tool that includes an assessment of the severity of illness and body mass index (BMI). This tool has also been shown to be valid and reliable in acute-care settings. Table 1.3 is a screening tool for use in inpatient adult populations (20,21). Figure 1.2 is another inpatient screen used in adult acute-care populations.

Table 1.2　Malnutrition Universal Screening Tool[a]

	Score
Step 1: BMI (kg/m^2)*	
20 (> 30 obese)	0
18.5–20	1
< 18.5	2
Step 2: % weight loss (unplanned in past 3–6 months)	
< 5	0
5–10	1
> 10	2
Step 3: If patient is acutely ill and has been or is likely to be without intake for > 5 days	2

Total score	Risk
0	Low
1	Medium
> 2	High

[a]If unable to obtain height and weight, see "MUST" Explanatory Booklet for alternative measurements and use of subjective criteria.

Adapted with permission from Malnutrition Advisory Group. Malnutrition Universal Screening Tool (MUST). British Association for Parenteral and Enteral Nutrition (BAPEN). Last update 2006. http://www.bapen.org.uk/must_tool.html. Accessed January 4, 2008.

Table 1.3　The Short Nutritional Assessment Questionnaire[a]

Question	Score
Did you lose weight unintentionally?	
> 6 kg in past 6 mo	3
> 3 kg in the past month	2
Did you experience a decreased appetite over the past month?	1
Did you use supplemental drinks or tube feeding over the past month?	1

[a]Patients who scored 0 or 1 points were classified as well-nourished and did not receive intervention. Patients who scored 2 points were classified as moderately malnourished and received nutritional intervention. Patients who scored 3 points were classified as severely malnourished and received nutritional intervention and treatment by a dietitian.

Reprinted with permission from Kruizenga HM, Van Tulder MW, Seidell JC, Thijs A, Ader HJ, Van Bokhorst-de van der Schueren MA. Effectiveness and cost-effectiveness of early screening and treatment of malnourished patients. *Am J Clin Nutr.* 2005;82:1082–1089.

Figure 1.2   Nutrition Screen Example

Nutrition Screening:
- ☐ **No risk factors**
- ☐ Outpatient handout given

Consult sent to Nutritional Services if one or more of the risk factors below are checked:
- ☐ Confused/unresponsive
- ☐ Eating less than half of usual food intake the past 7 days
- ☐ Unintentional weight change greater that 10 lbs/3months
- ☐ Pressure ulcers/nonhealing wounds (*consult sent to Enterostomal Therapist if applicable*)
- ☐ Tube feeding
- ☐ Home TPN

This nutrition screening form is part of the health screening form of Mount Carmel West Hospital, Columbus, Ohio.

Figure 1.3 is an example of a screening tool that was developed and validated for use with elderly patients/clients in community or long-term care settings (22,23). The Mini Nutritional Assessment—Short Form (MNA-SF) (not shown) is a brief screening tool that can be used to determine whether a more complete assessment using the entire Mini Nutritional Assessment (MNA) (Figure 1.3) is needed (22–24).

Figure 1.3   Mini Nutritional Assessment (MNA)®.

Nestlé Nutrition INSTITUTE   MINI NUTRITIONAL ASSESSMENT
MNA®

Date: _____
Last name: _____ First name: _____
Sex: _____   Age: _____
Weight, kg: _____ Height, cm: _____
I.D. Number: _____

Complete the screen by filling in the boxes with the appropriate numbers.
Add the numbers for the screen. If score is 11 or less, continue with the assessment to gain a Malnutrition Indicator Score.

Screening	
A	Has food intake declined over the past 3 months due to loss of appetite, digestive problems, chewing or swallowing difficulties? 0 = severe loss of appetite 1 = moderate loss of appetite 2 = no loss of appetite ☐
B	Weight loss during the last 3 months 0 = weight loss greater than 3 kg (6.6 lbs) 1 = does not know 2 = weight loss between 1 and 3 kg (2.2 and 6.6 lbs) 3 = no weight loss ☐
C	Mobility 0 = bed or chair bound 1 = able to get out of bed/chair but does not go out 2 = goes out ☐
D	Has suffered psychological stress or acute disease in the past 3 months 0 = yes 2 = no ☐

(continues next page)

Figure 1.3   Mini Nutritional Assessment (MNA)® (continued)

E	Neuropsychological problems	
	0 = severe dementia or depression	
	1 = mild dementia	
	2 = no psychological problems	☐

F	Body Mass Index (BMI) (weight in kg)/(height in m)^2	
	0 = BMI less than 19	
	1 = BMI 19 to less than 21	
	2 = BMI 21 to less than 23	
	3 = BMI 23 or greater	☐

Screening score (subtotal max. 14 points)   ☐ ☐

12 points or greater	Normal—not at risk—no need to complete assessment
11 points or below	Possible malnutrition—continue assessment

Assessment

G	Lives independently (not in a nursing home or hospital)	
	0 = no 1 = yes	☐

H	Takes more than 3 prescription drugs per day	
	0 = yes 1 = no	☐

I	Pressure sores or skin ulcers	
	0 = yes 1 = no	☐

J	How many full meals does the patient eat daily?	
	0 = 1 meal	
	1 = 2 meals	
	2 = 3 meals	☐

K	Selected consumption markers for protein intake	
	• At least one serving of dairy products (milk, cheese, yogurt) per day yes ☐ no ☐	
	• Two or more serving of legumes or eggs per week yes ☐ no ☐	
	• Meat, fish or poultry every day yes ☐ no ☐	

(continues next page)

Figure 1.3   Mini Nutritional Assessment (MNA)® (continued)

0.0	= if 0 or 1 yes
0.5	= if 2 yes
1.0	= if 3 yes

☐.☐

L Consumes two or more servings of fruits or vegetables per day?

0 = no   1 = yes   ☐

M How much fluid (water, juice, coffee, tea, milk ...) is consumed per day?

0.0 = less than 3 cups
0.5 = 3 to 5 cups
1.0 = more than 5 cups   ☐.☐

N Mode of feeding

0 = unable to eat without assistance
1 = self-fed with some difficulty
2 = self-fed without any problem   ☐

O Self view of nutritional status

0 = view self as being malnourished
1 = is uncertain of nutritional state
2 = views self as having no nutritional problem   ☐

P In comparison with other people of the same age, how does the patient consider his/her health status?

0.0 = not as good
0.5 = does not know
1.0 = as good
2.0 = better   ☐.☐

Q Mid-arm circumference (MAC) in cm

0.0 = MAC less than 21
0.5 = MAC 21 to 22
1.0 = MAC 22 or greater   ☐.☐

R Calf circumference (CC) in cm

0 = CC less than 31   1 = CC 31 or greater   ☐

(continues next page)

Figure 1.3   Mini Nutritional Assessment (MNA)® (continued)

Assessment (max. 16 points)   ☐ ☐.☐

Screening Score   ☐ ☐

Total Assessment (max. 30 points)   ☐ ☐.☐

Malnutrition Indicator Score		
17 to 23.5 points	at risk of malnutrition	☐
Less than 17 points	malnourished	☐

©Nestlé, 1994, Revision 2006. N67200 12/99/10M. For more information: www.mna-elderly.com. Reprinted with permission from ® Société des Produits Nestlé S.A., Vevey, Switzerland, Trademark Owners. References: Vellas B, Villars H, Abellan G, et al. Overview of the MNA®—its history and challenges. *J Nutr Health Aging.* 2006;10:456–465. Rubenstein LZ, Harker JO, Salva A, Guigoz Y, Vellas B. Screening for undernutrition in geriatric practice: developing the short-form Mini Nutritional Assessment (MNA-SF). *J Gerontol.* 2001;56A:M366-M377. Guigoz Y. The Mini Nutritional Assessment (MNA®) review of the literature—what does it tell us? *J Nutr Health Aging.* 2006;10466–487.

NUTRITION ASSESSMENT

Overview

Once the screening process has identified the potential that a nutrition problem exists, a nutrition assessment should be completed. As outlined in the NCP (see Chapter 7), nutrition assessment is the first step in providing nutrition care and uses information gathered during screening. Nutrition assessment incorporates more in-depth, comprehensive data, as well as data interpretation, to determine presence and extent of a nutrition problem. The exact data collected in the assessment vary, based on the practice setting, current individual/group clinical status, data needed to promote desired clinical outcomes, evidence-based recommendations, and whether it is an initial or follow-up assessment.

Five categories of nutrition assessment data—food/nutrition history, medical tests, laboratory data and procedures, client history, anthropometric data, and nutrition-focused physical examination—have been identified (25). The nutrition diagnostic language reference sheets (25) provide additional details. The nutrition assessment data are not only used for the initial assessment but are also repeatedly used throughout the NCP.

Box 1.2 illustrates the potential components used to assess nutritional status.

Accurate weight measurements are vital, because weight loss is felt to be strongly associated with adverse outcomes in some patient populations (26,27). The nutrition-focused physical examination provides an estimate of body composition and determination of presence of nutrient deficiency syndromes. In order to correctly diagnose nutrient deficiencies, an accurate estimation of recent intake is essential, along with evaluation of conditions that might alter nutrient digestion, absorption, utilization, and excretion (28–30).

Through the comprehensive nutrition assessment process, the RD can determine whether a nutrition diagnosis exists. Use of the assessment process may also help the RD determine the appropriate nutrition intervention to ameliorate the nutrition diagnosis. Monitoring and reevaluation are processes that are used for determining the effectiveness of the intervention. Appropriate documentation of the nutrition assessment is vital to ensure the delivery of optimal nutrition care.

Tools

The Subjective Global Assessment (SGA) (31) is a tool that uses findings of the history and physical examination to identify those patients who have signs and symptoms of global signs of malnutrition as well as physical changes associated with micronutrient deficiency (see Figure 1.4). It allows for accurate determination of nutritional status.

Box 1.2   Key Components of Nutrition Assessment

Food/Nutrition History
- Meal and snack patterns
- Adequacy of intake
- Food/nutrient tolerance
- Physical activity patterns
- Food availability

Client History
- Medical/surgical
- Medication/supplement usage
- Vital signs, history of current illness
- Socioeconomic status

Anthropometric Data
- Height
- Weight (current, usual, ideal)
- Body mass index (BMI)
- Waist-to-hip ratio
- Growth rate
- Rate of weight change

Medical Procedures, Laboratory Data, and Test Results
- Gastric emptying studies
- Bone scans
- Electrolytes
- Glucose/Hemoglobin A1C
- Lipid panel

Nutrition-Focused Physical Examination
- Overall musculature, adipose stores
- Oral (tongue, gums, lips, mucous membranes)
- General physical appearance

The SGA has been validated for use in several patient populations, although slight variations in the tool have been used.

Figure 1.4   Subjective Global Assessment

Subjective Global Assessment

A. History
  1. Weight change
     i) Overall loss in past 6 months: amount = #_____lb;
        % loss =_____
     ii) Change in past 2 weeks: ☐ increase   ☐ decrease
         ☐ no change

  2. Dietary intake change relative to normal
     i) No change_____
     ii) Change: _____ duration = _____ # weeks
        1. Suboptimal solid diet_____
        2. Full-liquid diet_____
        3. Hypocaloric liquids_____
        4. Starvation_____

  3. Gastrointestinal symptoms for more than 2 weeks
     i) None_____
     ii) Nausea_____
     iii) Vomiting_____
     iv) Diarrhea_____
     v) Anorexia_____

  4. Functional capacity
     i) No changes_____
     ii) Working suboptimally_____
     iii) Ambulatory_____
     iv) Bedridden_____

  5. Disease and its relation to nutritional requirements
     i) Primary diagnosis_____
     ii) Stress Level: none ___low ____moderate ____ high
         stress___

B. Physical Examination (for each trait specify: 0 = normal,
   1 = mild, 2 = moderate, 3 = severe)
  1. Loss of subcutaneous fat_____
  2. Muscle wasting (quadriceps, deltoids)_____

(continues next page)

Figure 1.4   Subjective Global Assessment (continued)

> 3. Ankle edema _____
> 4. Sacral edema_____
> 5. Ascites_____
>
> C. SGA Rating (select one)
> 1. A = Well-nourished ___
> 2. B = Moderately (or suspected of being) malnourished ___
> 3. C = Severely malnourished ___

Reprinted from Detsky AS, McLaughlin JR, Baker JP, Johnston N, Whittaker S, Mendelson RA, Jeejeebhoy KN. What is subjective global assessment of nutritional status? *JPEN J Parenter Enteral Nutr.* 1987;11:8–13, with permission from the American Society for Parenteral and Enteral Nutrition (A.S.P.E.N.). A.S.P.E.N. does not endorse the use of this material in any form other than its entirety.

Guidelines

The following are the key points to remember in the screening and assessment process:

- A policy must be in place to ensure nutritional risk screening in all health care settings (32).
- Patients admitted to an acute-care setting in the United States must be screened for nutritional risk within 24 hours of admission. It is not necessary that a dietetics professional complete this screen (32).
- The nutritional risk screen should be simple, quick, reliable, and efficient. The goal of screening should be to determine whether there is risk, not to quantify that risk.
- A policy must be in place to define which patients require nutrition assessment, when that assessment should take place, and which criteria are used to determine nutritional status (32).
- A policy must be in place to define when rescreening should occur. Time frames for assessment and

rescreening should consider the institution's average length of stay and patient population, not staffing requirements.

- All policies regarding screening and assessment should provide for consistent level of care regardless of weekends or holidays.

Joint Commission Standards Relating to Screening and Assessment

Standards (32)

- **PC.2.120:** The hospital defines in writing the time frames for conducting the initial assessment.
- **PC.2.130:** Initial assessments are performed as defined by the hospital.
- **PC.2.150:** Patients are re-assessed as needed.

Elements of Performance (32)

- **PC.2.120:** A nutrition screen, when warranted by the patient's needs or condition, is completed within no more than 24 hours of inpatient admission.
- **PC.2.130:** Each patient's initial assessment is conducted within the time frame specified by the needs of the patient, hospital policy, and law and regulations.

REFERENCES

1. Naber TH, Schermer T, de Bree A, Nusteling K, Eggink L, Kruimel JW, Bakkeren J, van Heereveld H, Katan MB. Prevalence of malnutrition in nonsurgical hospitalized patients and its association with disease complications. *Am J Clin Nutr.* 1997;66:1232–1239.
2. Keller HH. Malnutrition in institutionalized elderly: How and why? *J Am Geriatr Soc.* 1993;41:1212–1218.
3. McWhirter JP, Pennington CR. Incidence and recognition of malnutrition in hospital. *BMJ.* 1994;308:945–948.

4. Reilly JJ Jr, Hull SF, Albert N, Waller A, Bringardner S. Economic impact of malnutrition: a model system for hospitalized patients. *JPEN J Parenteral Enteral Nutr.* 1988;12:371–376.

5. Shulkin DJ, Kinosian B, Glick H, Glen-Puschett C, Daly J, Eisenberg JM. The economic impact of infections: an analysis of hospital costs and charges in surgical patients with cancer. *Arch Surg.* 1993;128:449–452.

6. Cederholm T, Jagren C, Hellstrom K. Outcome of protein-energy malnutrition in elderly medical patients. *Am J Med.* 1995;98:67–74.

7. Mullen JL, Buzby GP, Matthews DC, Smale BF, Rosato EF. Reduction of operative morbidity and mortality by combined preoperative and postoperative nutritional support. *Ann Surg.* 1980;192:604–613.

8. Robinson G, Goldstein M, Levine GM. Impact of nutritional status on DRG length of stay. *JPEN J Parenter Enteral Nutr.* 1987;11:49–51.

9. Hassell JT, Games AD, Shaffer B, Harkins LE. Nutrition support team management of enterally fed patients in a community hospital is cost-beneficial. *J Am Diet Assoc.* 1994;94:993–998.

10. Hedberg AM, Lairson DR, Aday LA, Chow J, Houston S, Wolf JA. Economic implications of an early postoperative enteral feeding protocol. *J Am Diet Assoc.* 1999;99:802–807.

11. Lacey K, Pritchett E. Nutrition care process and model: ADA adopts road map to quality care and outcomes management. *J Am Diet Assoc.* 2003;103:1061–1072.

12. American Dietetic Association. ADA's definitions for nutrition screening and nutrition assessment. *J Am Diet Assoc.* 1994;94:838–839.

13. Weinsier RL, Hunker EM, Krumdieck CL, Butterworth CE. Hospital malnutrition: a prospective evaluation of general medical patients during the course of hospitalization. *Am J Clin Nutr.* 1979;32:418–426.

14. Coats KG, Morgan SL, Bartolucci AA, Weinsier RL. Hospital-associated malnutrition: a reevaluation 12 years later. *J Am Diet Assoc.* 1993;93:27–33.

15. Singh H, Watt K, Vietch R, Cantor M, Duerksen DR. Malnutrition is prevalent in hospitalized medical patients: are house staff identifying the malnourished patient? *Nutrition.* 2006;22:350–354.

16. Ferguson M, Capra S, Bauer J, Banks M. Development of a valid and reliable malnutrition screening tool for adult acute hospital patients. *Nutrition.* 1999;15:458–464.

17. Stratton RJ, King CL, Stroud MA, Jackson AA, Elia M. "Malnutrition Universal Screening Tool" predicts mortality and length of hospital stay in acutely ill elderly. *Br J Nutr.* 2006;95:325–330.

18. ASPEN Board of Directors. *Clinical Pathways and Algorithms for Delivery of Parenteral and Enteral Nutrition Support in Adults.* Silver Spring, MD: ASPEN; 1998.

19. Malnutrition Advisory Group. Malnutrition Universal Screening Tool (MUST). British Association for Parenteral and Enteral Nutrition (BAPEN). Last update 2006. http://www.bapen.org.uk/must_tool.html. Accessed January 4, 2008.

20. Kruizenga HM, Seidell JC, Wierdsma NJ, Van Bokhorst-devan der Schueren MAE. Development and validation of a hospital screening tool for malnutrition: the short nutritional assessment questionnaire. *Clin Nutr.* 2005;24:75–82.

21. Kruizenga HM, Van Tulder MW, Seidell JC, Thijs A, Ader HJ, Van Bokhorst-de van der Schueren MA. Effectiveness and cost-effectiveness of early screening and treatment of malnourished patients. *Am J Clin Nutr.* 2005;82:1082–1089.

22. Guigoz Y, Vellas B, Garry PJ. Mini Nutritional Assessment. A practical assessment tool for grading the nutritional state of elderly patients. In Guigoz Y, Vellas B, Garry PJ, eds. *Facts and Research in Gerontology, Supplement 2.* New York, NY: Spraeger; 1994:15–59.

23. Rubenstein LZ, Jarker J, Guigoz Y, Vellas B. Comprehensive geriatric assessment (CGA) and the MNA: an overview of CGA, nutritional assessment, and development of a shortened version of the MNA. In: Vellas B, Garry PJ, Guigoz Y, eds. *Mini Nutritional Assessment (MNA): Research and Practice in the Elderly.* Nestlé Nutrition Workshop Series. Clinical & Performance Programme, vol. 1, Basel, Switzerland: Karger; 1997.

24. Cohendy R, Rubenstein LZ, Eledjam JJ: The Mini Nutritional Assessment-Short Form for preoperative nutritional evaluation of elderly patients. *Aging Clin Exp Res.* 2001;13:293–297.

25. *International Dietetics and Nutrition Terminology (IDNT) Reference Manual.* Chicago, IL: American Dietetic Association; 2008.

26. Dewys WD, Begg C, Lavin PT, Band PR, Bennett JM, Bertino JR, Cohen MH, Douglass HO Jr, Engstrom PF, Ezdinli EZ, Horton J, Johnson GJ, Moertel CG, Oken MM, Perlia C, Rosenbaum C, Silverstein MN, Skeel RT, Sponzo RW, Tormey DC. Prognostic effect of weight loss prior to chemotherapy in cancer patients. *Am J Med.* 1980;69:491–497.

27. Epstein AM, Read JL, Hoefer M. The relation of body weight to length of stay and charges for hospital services for patients undergoing elective surgery: a study of two procedures. *Am J Public Health.* 1987;77:993–997.

28. Sullivan DH, Sun S, Walls RC. Protein-energy undernutrition among elderly hospitalized patients: a prospective study. *JAMA.* 1999;281:2013–2019.

29. Tkatch L, Rapin CH, Rizzoli R, Slosman D, Nydegger V, Vasey H, Bonjour JP. Benefits of oral protein supplementation in elderly patients with fracture of the proximal femur. *J Am Coll Nutr.* 1992;11:519–525.

30. Larson J, Unosson M, Ek AC. Effect of dietary supplement on nutritional status and clinical outcome in 501 geriatric patients: a randomized study. *Clin Nutr.* 1990;9:179–184.

31. Detsky AS, McLaughlin JR, Baker JP, Johnston N, Whittaker S, Mendelson RA, Jeejeebhoy KN. What is subjective global assessment of nutritional status? *JPEN J Parenter Enteral Nutr.* 1987;11:8–13.

32. Joint Commission Board of Directors. *2007 Comprehensive Accreditation Manual for Hospitals.* Oak Brook, IL: Joint Commission; 2007.

chapter 2

Patient History

GAIL CRESCI, MS, RD, CNSD

The patient history elicits subjective information from the patient, his or her family, and/or caregivers. The patient history identifies nutrition issues at the time of the initial assessment; it is also useful in the monitoring phase of patient care. During this phase, patient history components can help assess whether the patient understands, tolerates, and complies with nutrition recommendations. Furthermore, the patient history may provide insight into why the patient's nutritional status is not improving despite nutrition interventions. Therefore, it is important to perform ongoing patient histories throughout the individual's continuum of care.

MEDICAL HISTORY

The patient's medical history should be reviewed closely to allow identification of factors that may influence nutritional status. Understanding the pathophysiology of various disease states, illnesses, surgeries, and medication interactions is necessary for noting factors that could put a patient at nutritional risk. Box 2.1 includes components for a detailed nutrition-oriented medical history (1–3). Tables 2.1, 2.2, and 2.3 present potential nutritional consequences after various gastrointestinal surgeries (1,4).

Box 2.1 Components of a Nutrition-Oriented Medical History

Chief Complaint
- Reason for seeking medical care (diagnosis)
- Includes onset and duration

Current Health Status
- Acute illness or injury
- Hydration status
- Infections, fever
- Open wounds, draining fistulas/abscesses
- Recent weight loss or gain greater than 10% of usual weight, time frame (≤ 6 months), stated vs documented, intentional vs unintentional, has weight stabilized or has patient continued to lose/gain?
- Usual body weight 20% more or less than ideal body weight
- Anorexia, nausea, vomiting, diarrhea, constipation, steatorrhea, heart burn, gastroesophageal reflux, abdominal pain
- Dysphagia—difficulty swallowing
- Functional status—recent change?

Chronic Disease States
- Carcinoma
- Cardiac disease
- Chronic lung disease
- Inflammatory bowel disease (eg, Crohn's disease, ulcerative colitis)
- Developmental delay
- Diabetes
- Epilepsy
- Hepatic disease
- Hyperlipidemia
- Peptic ulcer
- Renal disease
- Neurological disorders

Psychiatric History
- Depression
- Eating disorders
- Psychosis

Surgeries
- History of operations; any complications noted?
- Gastrointestinal tract resection or reconstruction

(continues next page)

Box 2.1   Components of a Nutrition-Oriented Medical History
(continued)

- Limb amputations restricting mobility, independence (adjust anthropometrics as needed)
- Organ transplants
- Postoperative infections
- Slow healing wounds/decubiti
- Enterocutaneous fistulas, ostomies

Diagnostic Procedures (for which prolonged NPO status is required)

Medical Therapies (dialysis, chemotherapy or radiation therapy, mechanical ventilation)

Family Health History
- Allergies (including food)
- Cancer
- Cardiovascular disease
- Diabetes
- Neuroendocrine disorders
- Food intolerances
- Genetic disorders that may affect nutritional status
- Gastrointestinal (GI) disorders
- Obesity
- Osteoporosis

Oral Health History
- Absence of teeth, poorly fitting dentures
- Difficulty chewing
- Mouth pain when eating
- Mouth sores

Medications
- Current prescriptions
- Over-the-counter medications
- Recent use of steroids, immunosuppressants, anticonvulsants
- Drug-nutrient interactions
- Drug-food interactions
- Nutrition supplements (vitamins/minerals, meal replacements)
- Complementary/alternative medicines
- Side effects that affect nutrient intake, nutrient absorption, excretion, and/or use

Table 2.1   Esophageal Surgery and Nutritional Consequences[a]

Type of Surgery	Potential Consequences
Resection/replacement	• Weight loss due to inadequate intake
Gastric pull-up	• Increased protein loss due to catabolism • Early satiety due to reduced reservoir capacity • Rapid emptying of hypertonic fluids
Colonic interposition	• May require enteral/parenteral nutrition until oral intake adequate • Anti-dumping diet; may malabsorb fat/fat-soluble vitamins, simple sugars, and various vitamins/minerals • Early satiety due to reduced reservoir capacity

[a]Note that consequences may occur only with extensive disease process and resection.

Table 2.2   Stomach Surgery and Nutritional Consequences[a]

Type of Surgery	Potential Consequences
Partial gastrectomy/vagotomy	• Early satiety due to reduced reservoir capacity • Delayed gastric emptying of solids due to stasis • Rapid emptying of hypertonic fluids • Achlorhydria may result in difficulty tolerating fibrous foods and malabsorption of vitamins and minerals (eg, vitamin B-12, iron)
Total gastrectomy	• Weight loss due to dumping/malabsorption, early satiety, anorexia, inadequate intake, unavailability of bile acids and pancreatic enzymes due to anastomotic changes • Achlorhydria may result in difficulty tolerating fibrous foods and malabsorption of vitamins and minerals (eg, vitamin B-12, iron) • Malabsorption may lead to anemia, metabolic bone disease, protein-calorie malnutrition • Bezoar formation • Vitamin B-12 deficiency due to lack of intrinsic factor

(continues next page)

Table 2.2   Stomach Surgery and Nutritional Consequences[a]
(continued)

Type of Surgery	Potential Consequences
Bariatric surgery (Vertical gastric banding, adjustable gastric banding, or roux-en-y gastric bypass)	• Protein-calorie malnutrition from malabsorption due to dumping; nonavailability of bile acids and pancreatic enzymes due to anastomotic changes • Dehydration, electrolyte abnormalities due to vomiting • Malabsorption of vitamins/minerals due to achlorhydria (vitamin B-12, iron); decreased absorptive surface and/or bypassed site of absorption (iron, vitamin B-12, folate, thiamine, Ca^{2+}); *or* decreased food intake • Bezoar formation

[a] Note that consequences may occur only with extensive disease process and resection.

Table 2.3   Intestinal Surgery and Nutritional Consequences[a]

Type of Surgery	Potential Consequences
Proximal	• Malabsorption of vitamins/minerals (Ca^{2+}, Mg^{2+}, folic acid, iron, vitamins A, D)
Distal	• Protein-calorie malnutrition due to malabsorption • Fat malabsorption • Malabsorption of fat-soluble vitamins (A, D, E, K) • Bacterial overgrowth, especially if ileocecal valve resected
Colon	• Fluid and electrolyte (K^+, Na^+, Cl^-) malabsorption • Decreased production of short-chain fatty acids

[a] Note that consequences may occur only with extensive disease process and resection.

MEDICATION HISTORY

It is common for patients to take multiple prescribed as well as over-the-counter medications, including alternative and herbal therapies. Food and medications can interact in many ways that can interfere with the medication's absorption and effectiveness. Often the active components of herbal therapies are unknown and could cause harm when taken with other medications. Many medications can also interfere with the ingestion, digestion, and absorption of nutrients. Individuals most at risk for drug-nutrient interactions are those receiving multiple medications, the chronically ill, and the elderly (5).

In recognition of this, the Joint Commission—formerly the Joint Commission on Accreditation of Healthcare Organizations (JCAHO)—endorses the importance of safe use of medications in providing nutrition intervention and education. Ideally, a multidisciplinary approach should be taken between the dietitian, pharmacist, physician, and nurse, to educate the patient on potential drug-nutrient interactions. Table 2.4 lists medications identified for inpatient and outpatient education for potential drug-nutrient interactions (6). Box 2.2 presents some potential nutrient and metabolic alterations caused by various medications (7).

Table 2.4 Medications That May Require Education on Potential Drug-Nutrient Interactions[a]

Drug	Interaction
Captopril	Food decreases bioavailability.
Ciprofloxacin	Complexation of drug with divalent and trivalent cations in enteral feedings; do not administer suspension with feeding tubes because of potential occlusion. With continuous enteral feedings, stop infusion for 2 hours before and 2 hours after quinolone if administered via the GI tract.
Amiodarone, amlodipine, atorvastatin, benzodiazepines, buspirone, carbamazepine, cilostazol, clomipramine, cyclosporine, diazepam, felodipine, indinavir, isradipine, lovastatin, methadone, nifedipine, nimodipine, nitrendipine, nisoldipine, saquinavir, sertraline, sildenafil, simvastien, sirolimus, tacrolimus, triazolam, verapamil	Grapefruit juice and dietary supplements that contain grapefruit bioflavonoids increase bioavailability because of inhibition of hepatic P-450 metabolism. Tangelos and Seville oranges may have a similar effect.
Griseofulvin	Take microsize forms with or after a high-fat meal or whole milk to increase absorption.
Levodopa	Dietary amino acids compete with drug for absorptive sites, decreasing bioavailability.

(continues next page)

Table 2.4 Medications That May Require Education on Potential Drug-Nutrient Interactions[a] (continued)

Drug	Interaction
Monoamine oxidase inhibitors	Avoid foods high in tyramine and other pressor amines to prevent hypertensive crisis.
Phenytoin	Decreased absorption with enteral feedings; hold enteral feedings 2 hr before and after dose.
Prednisone/dexamethasone	Long-term therapy may result in need for protein, calcium, potassium, phosphorus, folate, and vitamins A, C, and D supplementation.
Quinidine gluconate	Increased absorption on an empty stomach; may take with food or milk to decrease GI irritation; caution with increased potassium intake, as it may increase the drug's effects.
Tetracycline	Impaired absorption due to chelation if taken with iron-, calcium-, zinc-, and magnesium-rich foods.
Warfarin	Vitamin K decreases effectiveness; foods that make the urine acidic may decrease drug excretion; foods that make the urine basic may increase drug excretion.

[a]The registered dietitian should use clinical judgment regarding additional drug-nutrient interaction patient education.

Box 2.2   Drug-Induced Nutritional and Metabolic Alterations

Altered Taste
- Chemotherapeutic agents (carboplatin, cisplatin, etoposide, interferon alpha, teniposide)
- Sulfonylureas
- Disulfiram
- Captopril, metronidazole (Flagyl)—metallic taste

Appetite Changes
- *Increased:* Steroids, megestrol, androgens, benzodiazepines, antihistamines, insulin, phenothiazines, sulfonylureas
- *Decreased:* Antibiotics, antineoplastics, anticonvulsants, levodopa, thiazides, fluoxetine, amphetamines, weight loss products/appetite suppressants

Dry Mouth
- Radiation therapy, diuretics, antihistamines, tricyclic antidepressants, atropine-like drugs

Nausea/Emesis
- Antibiotics, thiazides, chemotherapeutic agents

Diarrhea
- Antibiotics, neomycin, prokinetic agents, cholinergics, cathartics, lactulose; enteral delivery of magnesium-containing medications, potassium-containing medications, hyperosmolar medications, sorbitol-containing medications

Constipation
- Barbiturates, vecuronium, opiates (morphine, codeine)

Hyperglycemia
- Steroids, theophylline, tacrolimus, chemotherapeutic agents (L-asparaginase, interferon, methotrexate)

Hypoglycemia
- Pentamidine, insulin, oral hypoglycemic agents

Altered Fat Metabolism/Absorption
- Cyclosporine, androgens, estrogen, progestin, cholestyramine, aluminum-containing antacids

(continues next page)

Box 2.2   Drug-Induced Nutritional and Metabolic Alterations
(continued)

Sodium Alterations
- *Loss:* Laxatives, diuretics, probenecid
- *Excess:* Penicillin G sodium, excessive delivery of normal saline

Potassium Alterations
- *Loss:* Diuretics, laxatives, probenecid, amphotericin B
- *Excess:* Spironolactone, tacrolimus, penicillin G potassium (reduced loss)

Phosphorus
- *Loss:* Binders (sucralfate, aluminum, calcium, magnesium, sevelamer [renagel]), corticosteroids, furosemide, thiazides
- *Excess*: Phosphorus-containing bowel preparation kits, several doses (eg, Fleets, Phospha-soda), especially for renal failure patients

Magnesium Alterations
- *Loss:* Diuretics, amphotericin B, ciprofloxacin, cyclosporine, probenecid, carbenicillin, pentamidine, cisplatin, tacrolimus
- *Excess*: Bowel preparation (milk of magnesia)

Calcium Loss
- Furosemide, triamterene, probenecid, corticosteroids, cisplatin, amphotericin B, calcitonin, phenytoin, pentamidine, mithramycin

---

SOCIAL HISTORY

A social history contains information regarding an individual's socioeconomic status, housing situation, access to a social support system, access to medical care, activity level, food purchasing and preparation capabilities, and religious practices. Understanding the social background allows the health care provider to tailor the nutrition care plan to better meet the patient's needs. Box 2.3 contains components of a detailed nutrition-oriented social history (2,3,8).

Box 2.3   Components of a Social History

Socioeconomic Status
- Employment status
- Income from Social Security, food stamps
- Government programs: Women, Infants and Children (WIC), Medicare, Medicaid, others
- Available food storage (eg, ± refrigeration (full-sized vs small "dorm sized," ice chest)
- Food delivery programs, such as Meals on Wheels

Housing Situation
- Lives alone
- Urban vs rural area
- Lives with family member, caregiver
- Lives in group home, skilled care facility, etc
- Prison
- Homeless

Social and Medical Support
- Family members
- Friends
- Access to medical care (Medicare, Medicaid, private medical insurance)

History of Recent Crisis
- Job loss
- Family member death
- Trauma, surgery
- Daily stress level

Activity Level
- Exercise (sedentary, moderately active, very active)
- House or bed-bound
- Ability to perform Activities of Daily Living
- Tremors (Parkinson's disease), seizure activity
- Posturing
- Seizure activity

(continues next page)

Box 2.3   Components of a Social History (continued)

Meal Preparation
- Who purchases and prepares foods? (eg, ability and skill to prepare food)
- Meal preparation facilities (full kitchen vs "hot plate," microwave)
- Shopping facilities (grocery store vs convenience markets); dining out

Other Factors
- Religious and cultural dietary practices
- Use of tobacco products
- Alcohol and drug use or abuse
- Support group attendance (weight control, substance abuse, etc)
- Home nutrition support therapy or nursing care

NUTRITION HISTORY

A nutrition history contains data regarding an individual's food habits, eating patterns, dietary restrictions, food intolerances, and identification of factors influencing nutrient intake. Components of a nutrition history are listed in Box 2.4 (8). Multiple methods can be used to obtain the dietary history including a 24-hour recall, food frequencies, and food records, logs, or diaries. In the hospital setting, calorie counts or direct observation for 24 to 72 hours may be used. Many advantages and disadvantages have been identified for each method (see Table 2.5) (2,8). The information obtained in a diet history may include qualitative or semiquantitative data. To increase the accuracy of the diet history, multiple methods are often used together. Boxes 2.5 through 2.8 list age-specific patient history questions for infants and children, adolescents, older adults, and pregnant women.

Box 2.4   Components of a Nutrition History

- Current diet order
- Current dietary habits (see Table 2.5)
- Days on clear liquids, inadequate intake, or nothing by mouth (NPO)
- Dietary restrictions (past and present)
- Recent dietary changes (intentional vs unintentional)
- Food consistency restrictions (soft, pureed, or liquid)
- Appetite assessment (poor, fair, good, or excellent)
- Satiety level
- Snack consumption
- Beverage consumption
- Alcohol consumption
- Food intolerances
- Food allergies
- Taste changes or aversions
- Ethnic, religious, and cultural dietary influences
- Fad diets
- Vitamin and mineral supplements
- Herbal supplements
- Commercial dietary supplements, protein powders, meal replacements, etc

Table 2.5 Methods for Obtaining a Diet History

Method	Description	Advantages	Disadvantages
24-hour recall	Food, beverage, and supplement consumption for the past 24 hours provided	• Simple, quick • Most patients can recall foods eaten • Reading and writing skills not required • Does not influence usual diet patterns	• Reliance on patient to accurately recall foods eaten and portion sizes • Interviewer must interpret portion sizes • May not be representative of usual intake
Food Frequency	Patient selects from a list which foods, beverages, and supplements are frequently consumed	• Can provide an overall evaluation of which nutrients are consumed over time • Easily standardized • Beneficial when used with 24-hour recall	• Requires patient to remember foods eaten • Does not give data on daily food portions or meal patterns • Reading and writing ability required unless patient is interviewed • Food list may not represent all foods patient eats

(continues next page)

Table 2.5 Methods for Obtaining a Diet History (continued)

Method	Description	Advantages	Disadvantages
Food diary/record	A 3- to 7-d record of all food, beverages, and supplements consumed; should include a weekend day	• Provides data about serving sizes, food preparation method, and time food eaten • Reduces error due to reliance on "recall"	• Large commitment for the patient • Requires reading and writing skills • Process itself may alter normal food consumption patterns • Recorder must be familiar with portion sizes
Nutrient intake record (calorie count)	Recording of actual nutrient consumption via direct observation or tray audit	• Visual observation of actual eating patterns rather than reliance on patient interpretation • Useful for hospitalized or long-term-care facility patients	• Usually subjective estimates of nutrient consumption by patient, nurses, family members • Observers usually poorly trained • Serving sizes may vary • Waiting for results is time consuming and may delay optimal nutrition intervention • Low priority and often overlooked and incomplete • Frequently inaccurate

**Box 2.5   Patient History Questions for Caregivers
of Infants and Children**

- What type of milk (eg, breast milk, cow's milk, soy milk, rice milk, [note fat content], or formula) are you feeding your child?
- How many times per day are you nursing?
- How much water and formula do you use in preparing your child's formula? How do you prepare formula?
- What water source do you use to prepare formula?
- How many ounces of formula or milk does your child drink each day?
- How many wet diapers does your child have per day?
- What else does your child drink during the day (eg, juice [100%?], soda, tea, water)?
- Do you put your child to bed with a bottle? What's in it?
- What solid foods does your child eat? When were these introduced in their diet?
- How many meals does your child eat per day?
- Does your child snack? If so, how often and what does it consist of?
- Does your child avoid any specific foods or food groups (eg, milk, meats, vegetables)?
- Does your child take any vitamin, mineral, iron, fluoride, or food supplements? If so, how often?
- Does your child ever chew on any nonfood items such as clay, dirt, paint chips, or woodwork?
- How old is your home? Does it have lead pipes or lead paint? Has the water ever been checked for lead? Are you renovating your home?

Box 2.6   Patient History Questions for Adolescents

- How many meals do you eat per day?
- Do you skip meals?
- How many meals are eaten away from home each day? Which ones? Where are they obtained?
- Who prepares meals at home?
- Are any specific foods or food groups avoided? Which ones and why?
- Do you consume milk or yogurt? What type and how much daily?
- Are you following any special diet? (*Evaluate compliance based on diet recall, etc*)
- If the teenager has diabetes mellitus, does he or she self-monitor blood glucose levels? How often? What are the results?
- In the past month have you observed any changes in your dietary intake? Your weight?
- Do you drink alcohol? Do you take any medications not prescribed by a physician? Quantity, frequency, duration?
- Does the teenager exhibit poor self-esteem or body image?
- Have you ever induced vomiting or taken diuretics or cathartics to lose weight or keep from gaining weight?
- Are you physically active? How often do you exercise? What type of exercise do you do? How long do you do the exercise? Are you tired when you finish exercising?
- Do you take any vitamin, mineral, herbal, or food supplements? If so, how often?

Box 2.7   Patient History Questions for Older Adults

- Where do you live and with whom?
- Are you physically active? Are you housebound? Describe daily activity.
- Who prepares your meals?
- Who does the food shopping?
- Do you follow any special dietary restrictions? If so, what?
- Do you consume alcohol or use tobacco products? If so, how much?
- What medications do you take? When do you take them? What do you take them with? Do you take any medications not prescribed by a physician?
- Do you take any vitamin, mineral, herbal, fiber, or food supplements? If so, which ones? How often and what quantity?
- Do you have trouble chewing or swallowing?
- Have you had any changes in bowel habits in the past 2 weeks? If so, how?
- Do you avoid any foods or food groups? If so, which ones?
- How much fluid do you drink each day? What do you drink?
- How many meals do you eat per day? How much of each meal do you consume?
- Have you lost or gained weight in the past month without trying?

Box 2.8   Patient History Questions for Pregnant Women

- Did you follow any special diet before pregnancy?
- How much weight have you gained? Are you happy with this weight gain?
- Do you take prenatal vitamins? How often?
- Do you take any iron supplements?
- Do you take calcium supplements?
- Do you have any food allergies? If so, to what?
- Do you have any nonfood cravings (eg, ice, dirt, cornstarch, clay, detergent)?
- Do you drink alcohol? If so, quantity, frequency, and duration?
- How many meals do you eat daily? How many snacks?
- Do you avoid any specific foods, such as fruits, milk or dairy products, vegetables, or meats?
- How much milk or yogurt do you drink/eat, and what type?
- Do you have diabetes? If yes:
    - What type do you have (type 1, type 2, gestational diabetes, prediabetes)?
    - Do you self-monitor your blood glucose levels? If so, what are your glucose levels?
- Do you have a history of gestational diabetes?
- Are you experiencing morning sickness? Feeling nauseated and/or vomiting throughout the day? How often?
- Are you nauseated or vomiting so that you are unable to eat certain foods? If so, which ones?

REFERENCES

1. Cresci G. Nutritional care of surgery patients. In: Williams S, ed. *Essentials of Nutrition and Diet Therapy*. 8th ed. St. Louis, MO: Mosby; 2003:549–569.

2. Russell MK, Mueller C. Nutrition screening and assessment. In: Gottschlich M, DeLegge M, Mattox T, Mueller C, Worthington P, eds. *The A.S.P.E.N. Nutrition Support Core Curriculum: A Case-Based Approach—The Adult Patient*. Silver Spring, MD: ASPEN; 2007: 163–186.

3. Hammond K. History and physical examination. In: Matarese L, Gottschlich M, eds. *Contemporary Nutrition Support Practice: A Clinical Guide*. Philadelphia, PA: WB Saunders; 1998:17–32.

4. Parrish CR, Krenitsky J, Willcutts K, Radigan A. Gastrointestinal disease. In: Gottschlich M, DeLegge M, Mattox T, Mueller C, Worthington P, eds. *The A.S.P.E.N. Nutrition Support Core Curriculum: A Case-Based Approach—The Adult Patient*. Silver Spring, MD: ASPEN; 2007: 508–539.

5. Brown R. Drug-nutrient interactions. In: Cresci G, ed. *Nutrition Support for the Critically Ill: A Guide to Practice*. Boca Raton, FL: Taylor & Francis; 2005:341–355.

6. Karch A. *2008 Lippincott's Nursing Drug Guide*. Philadelphia, PA: Lippincott Williams and Wilkins; 2008.

7. Rollins C. Drug-nutrient interactions. In: Gottschlich M, DeLegge M, Mattox T, Mueller C, Worthington P, eds. *The A.S.P.E.N. Nutrition Support Core Curriculum: A Case-Based Approach—The Adult Patient*. Silver Spring, MD: ASPEN; 2007:340–359.

8. Hopkins B. Assessment of nutritional status. In: Gottschlich M, Matarese L, Shronts E, eds. *Nutrition Support Dietetics: Core Curriculum*. Silver Spring, MD: ASPEN; 1993:15–70.

chapter 3

Nutrition-Focused Physical Assessment

M. Patricia Fuhrman, MS, RD, FADA, CNSD

The information obtained during a physical examination adds depth and a unique perspective to a comprehensive nutrition assessment. A nutrition-focused physical assessment combines the physical examination, vital signs, and anthropometrics with the information gathered from the patient's medical record, laboratory data, and interview, to determine the optimal nutrition care plan (1–9). Physical assessment skills are developed and maintained through continuous practice. Findings of a physical examination should be reported using a methodical listing of systems, so that no area is overlooked.

Remember that with privilege comes responsibility. Although it is important to obtain the information that will enhance and complete the nutrition care plan, it is equally important not to subject the patient to unnecessary procedures or discomfort. The information from a physical examination can be obtained by performing the examination or by reviewing the findings of another health care professional.

OVERVIEW OF THE PHYSICAL EXAMINATION

In doing the physical examination, follow a head-to-toe approach in a methodical manner, so that nothing is overlooked (see Box 3.1) (5). Refer to Figure 3.1 for the anatomy of the abdominal quadrants (2,3,7). Box 3.2 summarizes some fundamental obligations of the clinician who performs the assessment.

Box 3.1   Outline for Performing a Physical Examination

<table>
<tr><td colspan="2" align="center">General Survey</td></tr>
<tr><td>Overall appearance</td><td>Ability to communicate</td></tr>
<tr><td>Contractures</td><td>Surgical wounds, drains,</td></tr>
<tr><td>Body positioning</td><td>   ostomies</td></tr>
<tr><td>Body habitus</td><td>Feeding devices</td></tr>
<tr><td>Level of consciousness</td><td>Vascular access devices</td></tr>
<tr><td>Amputations</td><td></td></tr>
<tr><td colspan="2" align="center">Vital Signs</td></tr>
<tr><td>Blood pressure</td><td>Temperature (range during the</td></tr>
<tr><td>Radial pulse</td><td>   previous 24 hours)</td></tr>
<tr><td></td><td>Respiration</td></tr>
<tr><td colspan="2" align="center">Anthropometrics</td></tr>
<tr><td>Height</td><td>Skinfold thickness</td></tr>
<tr><td>Weight</td><td>Muscle mass and tone</td></tr>
<tr><td colspan="2" align="center">Skin</td></tr>
<tr><td>Color/pigmentation</td><td>Temperature</td></tr>
<tr><td>Scars/lesions</td><td>Turgor</td></tr>
<tr><td>Bruises</td><td>Vascularity</td></tr>
<tr><td>Edema</td><td>Ecchymosis</td></tr>
<tr><td>Moisture</td><td>Wounds/ulcers</td></tr>
<tr><td>Texture</td><td>Petechia</td></tr>
</table>

(continues next page)

Box 3.1   Outline for Performing a Physical Examination
(continued)

Nails

Color	Shape
Lesions	Texture
Size	Clubbing
Flexibility	Koilonychia

Head

Shape and symmetry	Temporal arteries
Temporal muscle wasting	Condition of scalp/hair
Tenderness	Masses

Eyes

Cornea	Sclera
Conjunctiva (can alert the clinician to signs of dehydration)	Xanthomas

Nose (Nares)

Exterior: shape, discharge, oxygen delivery, nasogastric suction and enteral feeding devices

Interior: patency, shape, deviated septum, polyps, discharge

Mouth: look for symmetry, lesions, color, moisture

Lips (can alert the clinician to signs of dehydration)	Palates
	Gag reflex
Mucosa	Gums
Dentition	Feeding and oxygen devices
Tongue	Ability to chew and swallow

Neck

Trachea and thyroid	Tracheostomy
Parotid gland	Range of motion
Symmetry	Feeding devices

(continues next page)

Box 3.1 Outline for Performing a Physical Examination
(continued)

Chest: Cardiovascular and Respiratory Systems

Muscular and respiratory
 development

Edema

Auscultate for breath and heart
 sounds

Muscle wasting

IV access devices

Abdomen

Color

Contour/muscle development

Symmetry

Umbilicus

Scars/wounds

Ostomies

Feeding devices

Auscultate for bowel sounds

Palpate for distention, firmness,
 and tenderness

Musculoskeletal: Arms and Legs

Size/shape

Involuntary movements

Symmetry

Amputations

Strength

Range of motion

Joint pain

Muscle loss

Hair distribution

Skin discoloration

Swelling/edema

Neurological

Gross/fine motor skills

Mental acuity

Paralysis

Coordination

Weakness

Posturing

Seizures

Adapted with permission from Hammond KA, Hillhouse J. *Study Guide Nutrition-Focused Physical Assessment Skills for Dietitians.* Chicago, IL: American Dietetic Association; 1998:10–11.

Box 3.2   Responsibilities of Performing Physical Assessment

Practice universal precautions:
- Wash hands and clean equipment thoroughly between patients.
- Wear protective clothing whenever indicated.

Respect the patient's privacy and comfort:
- Inform the patient why the examination is being performed and by whom.
- Make the patient as comfortable as possible.
- Allow the patient to empty his bladder before examining the abdomen.
- Keep the patient's body covered except for the area being examined.

Communicate abnormal findings to the nurse or physician.

Figure 3.1   Abdominal Quadrants

The Abdominal Quadrants

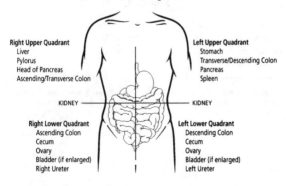

Right Upper Quadrant
Liver
Pylorus
Head of Pancreas
Ascending/Transverse Colon

Left Upper Quadrant
Stomach
Transverse/Descending Colon
Pancreas
Spleen

KIDNEY — — KIDNEY

Right Lower Quadrant
Ascending Colon
Cecum
Ovary
Bladder (if enlarged)
Right Ureter

Left Lower Quadrant
Descending Colon
Cecum
Ovary
Bladder (if enlarged)
Left Ureter

Source: Data are from references 2, 3, and 7.

VITAL SIGNS

The vital signs examination should be performed in a quiet environment (Table 3.1) (2,3,8). The patient should be rested, with no caffeine or smoking for at least 30 minutes before the measurement.

Table 3.1 Vital Signs

Vital Sign	Technique	Normal/Abnormal	Effect on Care Plan
Blood pressure	• Allow patient to rest at least 5 min before measuring • If abnormal, recheck later during the examination to verify	*Normal* • < 130 mm Hg systolic • < 85 mm Hg diastolic *Abnormal* • Hypertension: > 140 mmHg/90 mmHg • Orthostatic hypotension: rapid drop of 25 mm Hg when changing from supine to sitting or standing	• Orthostatic hypotension is associated with hypovolemia • Diet therapy may be appropriate for hypertension • Diet/herbal supplements can affect blood pressure (ie, yohimbe bark, ma huang/ephedra)
Radial pulse	• Count pulsations for 15 seconds and multiply by 4. • If irregular, count for 60 seconds	*Normal:* 60–100 pulses/min • Bradycardia: < 60/min • Tachycardia: > 100/min	• Tachycardia associated with hypovolemia and caffeine • Bradycardia associated with athletes and starvation

(continues next page)

Table 3.1   Vital Signs (continued)

Vital Sign	Technique	Normal/Abnormal	Effect on Care Plan
Respiration	• Count number of respirations while holding pulse, so patient is unaware of monitoring	*Normal:* 14–20 breaths/min	• Labored breathing/COPD can increase energy expenditure • Humidified air reduces insensible fluid loss
Temperature	Avoid hot/cold beverages for 10–15 min before measurement	Diurnal variation 35.8° to 37.3°C (96.4° to 99.1°F)	• Febrile • Increased caloric expenditure • Hypothermia or hyperthermia may indicate presence of inflammatory response

Source: Data are from references 2, 3, and 8.

47

EVALUATING HYDRATION STATUS

Refer to Tables 3.2 and 3.3 for parameters for evaluating under- and overhydration (1–3, 5, and 8).

Table 3.2   Underhydration (Fluid Deficit)

Clinical Presentation	*Possible Etiologies*
Vital sign aberrations	*Inadequate fluid intake*
• Decreased blood pressure	• IV fluids
• Decreased cardiac output	• Oral fluid intake
• Decreased central venous pressure	• Tube feeding flushes
• Decreased pulmonary artery wedge pressure	*Excessive losses*
• Increased heart rate	• Diaphoresis
• Increased temperature	• Diarrhea/emesis
• Increased systemic vascular resistance	• NG/fistula/drains/ostomy
Physical findings	• Dialysis, hemofiltration
• Input < output	• Persistent fevers
• Decreased weight	• Wounds, burns, paracentesis
• Sunken, dry eyes	• Hemorrhage
• Dark-colored urine, oliguria	• Polyuria
• Dry mucous membranes	• Medications
• Sticky saliva	• Anabolism
• Poor skin turgor	
• Cool, pale, clammy skin	
• Jugular vein flattened (< 3 cm when flat or lying down)	
Laboratory data	
• Elevated sodium	
• Elevated chloride	
• Elevated BUN	
• Elevated creatinine	
• Elevated hemoglobin	
• Elevated hematocrit	
• Elevated serum osmolality	
• Elevated urine-specific gravity	
Mental effects	
• Dizziness	
• Confusion	

Source: Data are from references 1–3, 5, and 8.

Table 3.3   Overhydration (Fluid Excess)

Clinical Presentation	Possible Etiologies
Vital-sign aberrations	*Excessive fluid intake*
• Increased blood pressure	• Surgical procedures
• Increased cardiac output	• IV fluids
• Increased central venous pressure	
• Increased pulmonary artery wedge pressure	*Interstitial fluid retention*
	• Hypoalbuminemia
Physical findings	*Disease processes*
• Input > output	• Renal failure
• Increased weight	• Liver failure, ascites
• Puffy, swollen eyes	• Congestive heart failure
• Light-colored urine	• Syndrome of inappropriate antidiuretic hormone (SIADH)
• Moist skin	• Severe hypertension
• Edema (peripheral and sacral)	
• Anasarca	
• Shortness of breath, dyspnea, lung crackles	
• Jugular vein distention (> 3 cm when sitting up)	

Source: Data are from references 1–3, 5, and 8.

PHYSICAL EXAMINATION TECHNIQUES

Inspection

Inspection is the most often used technique, yet the most difficult to master. See Table 3.4 for more information (1–9).

Table 3.4 Physical Examination Techniques: Inspection

Technique	Examples of Information Obtained			
	Body Composition	Nutritional Adequacy	Disease Process	Other
• Use sight, smell, and hearing. • Observe texture, size, color, and shape. • Perform in well-lighted areas.	• Obesity • Cachexia • Fluid status	• Skin integrity • Wound healing • Feeding devices	• Jaundice • Ascites • Fluid status	• Functional capacity • Mental status

Source: Data are from references 1–9.

Palpation and Percussion

Deep palpation and percussion are not always used in nutrition-focused examinations. However, it is important to know what sounds mean when reported by other health care professionals. Refer to Tables 3.5 and 3.6 for more on these techniques (1–9).

Table 3.5   Physical Examination Techniques: Palpation

Technique	*Examples of Information Obtained*
• Use palms and fingertip pads of hands • Use sense of touch • Feel vibrations and pulsations • Light palpation assesses pulse (jugular, radial, pedal) • Deep palpation assesses body structures • Palpate tender areas last. Avoid deep palpation of tender areas.	• Areas of tenderness • Muscle rigidity and distention • Fluid retention, pitting edema • Abdominal masses and girth • Skin integrity and moisture • Body temperature • Guarding or rebound tenderness with palpation may indicate peritonitis, perforation, etc

Source: Data are from references 1–9.

Table 3.6   Physical Examination Techniques: Percussion

	Examples of Information Obtained	
Technique	*Abdomen*	*Lungs*
• Use fingertip pads • Assess sounds to identify organ border, position, and shape • Requires practice and acute listening skills	• Tympany suggests obstruction • Dullness suggests ascites	• Dullness suggests fluid/tissue in place of air

Source: Data are from references 1–9.

Auscultation

To conduct an auscultation:
- Use naked ear or stethoscope
- Reduce extraneous noise
- Ask patient not to speak
- Place stethoscope lightly on the skin.

Specific methods for bowel auscultation are described in Table 3.7. See Table 3.8 for information specific to the auscultation of heart and lungs (1–9).

Table 3.7   Physical Examination Techniques: Auscultation of the Bowel

Technique	Examples of Information Obtained	Comments
• Listen for 3–5 min in RLQ (right lower quadrant); this is location of ileocecal valve. • If nothing is heard, listen for 1–2 min in other 3 quadrants. • Be patient. It could take 10 min to listen effectively to all 4 quadrants.	*Normal:* • Gurgling, high-pitched, every 5–15 seconds *Hypoactive:* • Quieter, every 15–20 seconds • Paralytic ileus or peritonitis *Hyperactive:* • Continuous, high-pitched, tinkling • Diarrhea, intestinal obstruction *Absent:* • Nothing after listening for 5 min in RLQ and 2 min in other 3 quadrants.	• Absence of bowel sounds is not always a contraindication to enteral feeding. • Bowel sounds signify the passage of air and fluid. Peristalsis may still occur in the absence of bowel sounds. • Presence of bowel sounds does not guarantee successful feeding.

Source: Data are from references 1–9.

**Table 3.8   Physical Examination Techniques:
Auscultation of Heart and Lungs**

	Technique	Examples of Information Obtained
Heart	Listen for normal "lub-dub"	Listen at 6 points of chest for: • Rhythm • Murmurs • Pericardial friction rub
Lungs	Listen for abnormal breath sounds	Continuous "musical" sounds: • Wheezing • Rhoncus • Pleural friction rub Discontinuous "brief" sounds: • Crackles

Source: Data are from references 1–9.

CLINICAL INTERPRETATION OF PHYSICAL EXAMINATION FINDINGS

When interpreting physical examination findings, it is important to note that an isolated nutrient deficiency is rarely found. Always consider possible nonnutritional causes. Signs and symptoms of a deficiency occur after prolonged diet inadequacy. Findings should be correlated with diet history and medical condition (10).

Eyes

In an eye examination, the following indicate normal health:

- Bright, clear, shiny, smooth cornea
- Pink and moist membranes
- Normal eye movement to follow objects

Table 3.9 lists clinical findings that may indicate nutritional deficiencies (10).

Table 3.9   Clinical Interpretation of Eye Examination Findings

Clinical Findings	Suspected Deficiency	Other Potential Etiologies
• Pale conjunctiva	• Iron	• Nonnutritional anemia
• Night blindness	• Vitamin A	• Heredity • Eye diseases
• Bitot's spots	• Vitamin A	
• Xerosis	• Vitamin A	• Aging • Allergies
• Redness, fissuring in corners of eyes	• Riboflavin • Pyridoxine	
• Ophthalmoplegia	• Thiamin • Phosphorus	• Brain lesion

Adapted with permission from Morrison SG. Clinical nutrition physical examination. *Support Line*. 1997;19(2):16–18. Copyright *Support Line*; DNS, a dietetic practice group of American Dietetic Association.

Hair

In an examination of a patient's hair, the following indicate normal health:

- Shiny, firm, not easily plucked
- Normal-appearing or thick
- Normal-appearing hair shaft and emergence from skin

Table 3.10 lists clinical findings that may indicate nutritional deficiencies (10).

Table 3.10   Clinical Interpretation of Hair Examination Findings

Clinical Findings	Suspected Deficiency	Other Potential Etiologies
• Flag sign • Easily plucked with no pain	• Protein • Seen in kwashiorkor and occasionally marasmus	• Overprocessing hair, as in excess bleaching
• Sparse	• Protein • Biotin • Zinc	• Alopecia from aging, chemotherapy, or radiation to the head • Endocrine disorders
• Corkscrew hair • Unemerged, coiled hairs	• Vitamin C	

Adapted with permission from Morrison SG. Clinical nutrition physical examination. *Support Line*. 1997;19(2):16–18. Copyright *Support Line*; DNS, a dietetic practice group of American Dietetic Association.

Nails

Uniform, rounded, and smooth nails are an indication of normal health. Table 3.11 lists clinical findings that may indicate nutritional deficiencies (10).

Table 3.11   Clinical Interpretation of Nail Examination Findings

Clinical Findings	Suspected Deficiency	Other Potential Etiologies
Transverse ridging	Protein	
Koilonychia	Iron	Considered normal if seen on toenails only

Adapted with permission from Morrison SG. Clinical nutrition physical examination. *Support Line*. 1997;19(2):16–18. Copyright *Support Line*; DNS, a dietetic practice group of American Dietetic Association.

Skin

When examining skin, uniform color, smoothness, and a healthy appearance are signs of normal health. Table 3.12 lists clinical findings that may indicate nutritional deficiencies (10).

Table 3.12   Clinical Interpretation of Skin Examination Findings

Clinical Findings	Suspected Deficiency	Other Potential Etiologies
• Scaling • Nasolabial seborrhea	• Vitamin A • Zinc • Riboflavin • Essential fatty acids • Pyridoxine	• Vitamin A excess • Nasal congestion
• Petechiae, especially perifollicular	• Vitamin C	• Abnormal blood clotting • Severe fever • Red spots from flea bite
• Purpura	• Vitamin C • Vitamin K	• Warfarin • Injury • Thrombocytopenia • Excessive vitamin E
• Follicular hyperkeratosis	• Vitamin A • Vitamin C	
• Pigmentation • Desquamation of sun-exposed areas	• Niacin	
• Cellophane appearance	• Protein	• Aging process
• Yellow pigmentation of palms of hands with normal white sclera	• Excess beta carotene	
• Body edema • Round, swollen face (moon face)	• Protein • Thiamin	• Medications, especially steroids
• Poor wound healing • Decubitus ulcers	• Protein • Vitamin C • Zinc • Kwashiorkor	• Poor skin care • Diabetes • Steroid use
• Pallor • Fatigue	• Iron	• Blood loss

Adapted with permission from Morrison SG. Clinical nutrition physical examination. *Support Line*. 1997;19(2):16–18. Copyright *Support Line*; DNS, a dietetic practice group of American Dietetic Association.

Oral Health

In an oral examination, the following are indicators of normal health:

- Lips smooth without sores
- Tongue red without swelling
- Normal surface
- Normal taste and smell
- Normal gums and teeth

Table 3.13 lists clinical findings that may indicate nutritional deficiencies (10).

Table 3.13   Clinical Interpretation of Oral Examination Findings

Clinical Findings	Suspected Deficiency	Other Potential Etiologies
• Cheilosis • Angular stomatitis	• Riboflavin • Pyridoxine • Niacin	• Excessive salivation due to ill-fitting dentures • Dry skin (winter) • Dehydration
• Atrophic lingual papillae	• Riboflavin • Niacin • Folate • Vitamin B-12 • Protein • Iron	
• Hypoguesia • Hyposmia	• Zinc	• Medications such as antineoplastic agents or sulfonylureas • Nasal congestion
• Mottled tooth enamel		• Excess fluoride
• Eroded enamel		• Suspect bulimia
• Cavities • Missing teeth		• Poor dental hygiene
• Retracted gums		• Periodontal disease
• Swollen, bleeding gums • Retracted gums with teeth	• Vitamin C	• Poor oral hygiene • Pregnancy

Adapted with permission from Morrison SG. Clinical nutrition physical examination. *Support Line*. 1997;19(2):16–18. Copyright *Support Line*; DNS, a dietetic practice group of American Dietetic Association.

Neurological Health and Other Clinical Findings of Note

Indicators of normal neurological health include the following:

- Psychological stability
- Normal reflexes and sensations

Table 3.14 lists clinical findings in a neurological examination that may indicate nutritional deficiencies (10). Table 3.15 summarizes selected other clinical findings of note (10).

Table 3.14   Clinical Interpretation of Neurologic Examination Findings

Clinical Findings	Suspected Deficiency	Other Potential Etiologies
• Dementia	• Niacin • Vitamin B-12	• Disease or age related • Increased calcium • Medications • Aluminum toxicity
• Confabulation • Disorientation	• Thiamin (Korsakoff's psychosis)	
• Foot and wrist drop	• Thiamin	
• Peripheral neuropathy with weakness and paresthesias • Ataxia and decreased tendon reflexes, fine tactile vibrator and position sense	• Thiamin • Pyridoxine • Vitamin B-12	
• Tetany	• Calcium • Magnesium • Vitamin D	

Adapted with permission from Morrison SG. Clinical nutrition physical examination. *Support Line*. 1997;19(2):16–18. Copyright *Support Line*; DNS, a dietetic practice group of American Dietetic Association.

Table 3.15   Clinical Interpretation of Other Examination Findings

Clinical Findings	Suspected Deficiency	Other Potential Etiologies
• Parotid enlargement • Hepatomegaly	• Protein • Bulimia	• Disease of the parotid or liver • Excess vitamin A
• Rickets or osteomalacia	• Vitamin D	

Adapted with permission from Morrison SG. Clinical nutrition physical examination. *Support Line*. 1997;19(2):16–18. Copyright *Support Line*; DNS, a dietetic practice group of American Dietetic Association.

REFERENCES

1. Pesce-Hammond K, Wessel J. Nutrition assessment and decision making. In: Merritt R, ed, *The A.S.P.E.N. Nutrition Support Practice Manual*, 2nd ed. Silver Springs, MD: American Society for Parenteral and Enteral Nutrition; 2006:3–37.

2. Bates B, ed. *A Guide to Physical Examination and History Taking*. 6th ed. Philadelphia, PA: JB Lippincott; 1995.

3. Elkin MK, Perry AG, Potter PA, eds. *Nursing Interventions and Clinical Skills*. St. Louis, MO: Mosby; 1996.

4. Hammond K. Nutrition-focused physical assessment. *Support Line*. 1996;18(4):1–4.

5. Hammond K, Hillhouse J. *Study Guide Nutrition-Focused Physical Assessment Skills for Dietitians*. Chicago, IL: American Dietetic Association; 1998.

6. Goff K. Assessment of the gastrointestinal tract. *Support Line*. 1997;19(2):3–7.

7. Hammond K. History and physical exam. In: Matarese LE, Gottschlich MM, eds. *Contemporary Nutrition Support Practice: A Clinical Guide*. 2nd ed. Philadelphia, PA: Saunders; 2003:14–44.

8. Murphy LM, Bickford V. Physical assessment of cardiopulmonary system: nutritional implication. *Support Line*. 1997;19(2):8–11.

9. Touger-Decker R, Sirois DA. Physical assessment of the oral cavity. *Support Line*. 1996;18(5):1–6.

10. Morrison SG. Clinical nutrition physical examination. *Support Line*. 1997;19(2):16–18.

chapter 4

Laboratory Assessment

CHERYL W. THOMPSON, PhD, RD, CNSD

Accurate interpretation of laboratory data requires knowledge of the appropriate test to order as well as nutritional and nonnutritional factors that alter blood chemistries. A complete diet history, including supplement usage and physical signs/symptoms, can provide important supportive information. Nonnutritional factors, such as disease processes, treatments, procedures, medications, and hydration status, can profoundly alter blood and urine chemistries and must be considered. Blood levels can also be carefully controlled by homeostatic mechanisms and may not reflect tissue stores. Ideally, any nutrition lab test ordered should evaluate tissue stores or nutrient function.

Keep in mind:

- A review of serial laboratory data is recommended. The direction and speed of change are more important than a static value.
- Assay methods vary greatly. Use reference values established by your laboratory.
- An improvement in nutrition parameters does not always confer clinical benefit. Improved clinical outcome remains the ultimate goal.
- Treat the patient, not the laboratory value. Abnormal laboratory reports that are unexpected or inconsistent

with the clinical picture should be repeated before treatment.

Laboratory data can be a critical component of each step in the Nutrition Care Process but must be interpreted carefully (see Box 4.1) (1). The Nutrition Care Process is covered in detail in Chapter 7.

Box 4.1   The Nutrition Care Process and Model and Laboratory Assessment

Step 1: Nutrition Assessment

- Evaluating nutritional status
- Screening for conditions such as diabetes or malabsorption

Step 2: Nutrition Diagnosis

- Diagnosing nutrition problems (eg, impaired nutrient utilization; altered nutrition-related laboratory values; and inadequate or excessive protein, carbohydrate, fat, vitamins, or minerals)
- Determining the etiology (causative or contributing factors)
- Identifying signs (defining characteristics)

Step 3: Nutrition Intervention

- Planning appropriate and measurable goals for control and/or improvement

Step 4: Nutrition Monitoring and Evaluation

- Reviewing progress toward goals (such as increasing or decreasing lab values)
- Monitoring the response to medical nutrition therapy
- Estimating risk of morbidity and/or mortality

HEPATIC TRANSPORT PROTEIN ASSESSMENT

Serum Proteins (2–6)

Despite the most advanced laboratory tests available for nutrition assessment, there is no single test that is both sensitive and specific for protein-calorie malnutrition. Evaluation of serum albumin, transferrin, and prealbumin requires simultaneous evaluation of nutrient intake, physical findings, and clinical condition, and must be interpreted with an awareness of their limitations. For example, during illness, nonnutritional factors alter serum protein concentrations, and changes cannot be interpreted as resulting from nutritional status or intake. Therefore, serum proteins have limited clinical utility during nutrition assessment and monitoring in acute-care settings, except in the evaluation of severity of illness.

Acute-Phase Response

The acute-phase response is a systemic response to acute or chronic inflammation associated with conditions such as infection, trauma, surgery, and cancer. Mediators, such as cytokines, are released that cause the liver to reprioritize the synthesis of proteins to those most critical for host defense and adaptive capabilities. Increased protein degradation and transcapillary losses also occur. Therefore, the serum concentrations of some proteins will increase while others decrease. An acute-phase response increases the C-reactive protein concentration, along with other positive acute-phase reactants like ceruloplasmin, ferritin, and others, while simultaneously decreasing albumin, transferrin, prealbumin, and retinol-binding protein. Regardless of nutrition support, these protein levels will not return to normal until the inflammatory stress subsides.

An elevated temperature and/or white blood cell count can be general indications of an inflammatory response. In addition, an increased C-reactive protein concentration or erythrocyte sedimentation rate (ESR) can be helpful in quantifying the intensity of an acute-phase response. C-reactive protein is not used as a nutritional parameter; however, it is often used to monitor the presence, intensity, and recovery from an inflammatory process. Simultaneous evaluation of the C-reactive protein may help to determine whether serum proteins are reduced because of an inflammatory process. Nevertheless, the routine practice is not warranted and additional costs must be considered, especially when multiple measurements are necessary to evaluate a trend (5). The C-reactive protein is most useful if there is no clinical indication of inflammatory response, but serum protein levels remain low despite what is thought to be adequate nutrient intake.

Albumin

In unstressed starvation, normal albumin levels are preserved because of decreased catabolism and increased mobilization of the body's extravascular stores (where approximately 60% of the body's albumin pool is found) (4).

In hospitalized patients, serum albumin is often misinterpreted as a nutritional marker. Albumin is neither sensitive to, nor specific for, acute protein malnutrition or the response to nutrition therapy. During a critical illness, factors that alter serum albumin include the acute-phase response, hydration (intravascular volume) status, disease state, clinical condition, and leakage of albumin from intravascular to extravascular spaces. Blood loss and perioperative fluid resuscitation will also contribute to rapid decreases in postoperative albumin levels. One consequence of hypoalbuminemia is a reduction in colloid osmotic pressure, with a corresponding shift of intravascular fluid into extravascular spaces, which may be evident as edema or ascites (4).

Albumin can be of use as a prognostic indicator of morbidity, mortality, and severity of illness, because serum concentrations are inversely correlated with inflammatory processes. Hypoalbuminemia has been associated with increased hospital length of stay, morbidity (eg, postoperative complications, infection, organ dysfunction), and mortality in numerous studies (3,6). Therefore, as an index of the severity of underlying disease, a low albumin can indirectly identify high-risk patients who may benefit most from nutrition assessment and early intervention (see Table 4.1).

Table 4.1   Factors That Decrease or Increase Albumin

Albumin	Factors That Decrease Albumin	Factors That Increase Albumin

Normal: 3.5–5.0 g/dL
Depletion:
  Mild: 3.0–3.4 g/dL
  Moderate: 2.4–2.9 g/dL
  Severe: < 2.4 g/dL
Half-life approximately 14–20 d
	• Acute-phase response[a]
	• Severe liver failure
	• Redistribution: intravascular volume overload, third spacing, pregnancy, minor decrease with recumbency
	• Increased losses: nephrotic syndrome, burns, protein-losing enteropathies, exudates
	• Severe zinc deficiency
		• Intravascular volume depletion
		• Intravenous albumin or plasminate, blood transfusions (temporary rise)
		• Anabolic steroids, possibly glucocorticoids

[a]Acute-phase response occurs with inflammation associated with conditions such as infection, injury, surgery, and cancer.

Transferrin

Compared to albumin, transferrin has a smaller and primarily intravascular body pool and shorter half-life. Although transferrin concentrations are reduced in severe protein-calorie malnutrition, they may be variable in mild to moderate degrees of malnutrition and overall lack of sensitivity and specificity to assess or monitor protein status.

The primary function of transferrin is to bind and transport iron. Therefore, synthesis of transferrin is inversely correlated with the body's iron stores. An elevated transferrin concentration often indicates early iron deficiency. It is also the last laboratory value to return to normal when iron deficiency is corrected. In addition to iron status, an awareness of the acute-phase response must be considered, because transferrin levels will decrease during acute illness (see Table 4.2).

Table 4.2   Factors That Decrease or Increase Transferrin

Transferrin	Factors That Decrease Transferrin	Factors That Increase Transferrin

Normal: 200–400 mg/dL
Depletion:
  Mild: 150–200 mg/dL
  Moderate: 100–149 mg/dL
  Severe: < 100 mg/dL
Half-life approximately 8–10 d
	• Acute-phase response
	• Chronic or end-stage liver disease
	• Uremia
	• Protein-losing states: some nephrotic syndromes, burns
	• Intravascular volume overload
	• High-dose antibiotic therapy (such as amino-glycosides, tetracycline, and some cephalosporins)
	• Iron overload
	• Severe zinc deficiency, protein calorie malnutrition
		• Iron deficiency, chronic blood loss
		• Pregnancy (markedly increases in 3rd trimester)
		• Intravascular volume depletion
		• Acute hepatitis
		• Oral contraceptives, estrogen

Although direct measurement of serum transferrin is more accurate, several equations are available to calculate transferrin from the total iron-binding capacity (TIBC). Depending on which equation is used, the calculated transferrin concentration can vary greatly. Verify with the laboratory which equation is most closely correlated with their assay methods.

Prealbumin (Transthyretin, Thyroxin-Binding Prealbumin)

Prealbumin is a carrier protein for thyroxin (thyroid hormone) and, combined with retinol-binding protein, transports vitamin A. Compared with albumin or transferrin, it has a shorter half-life, a smaller plasma pool, is influenced less by intravascular fluid volume, and is not affected as early or as significantly with liver disease. Therefore, it is often thought to be a more sensitive marker for protein and/or calorie deficiency. This sensitivity means that it is more likely to be a reflection of recent dietary intake than an accurate indicator of nutritional status. Although prealbumin has been used as a screening tool, its limitations must be considered, and it lacks adequate specificity to be effective as a sole criterion of malnutrition. Cost and lack of specificity and sensitivity limit its usefulness as a screening or assessment tool.

Prealbumin is known to decline rapidly with an acute-phase response and therefore is subject to similar limitations in interpretation as albumin and transferrin. Failure of pre-albumin to return to normal despite adequate protein and calories may indicate a sustained acute-phase response and/or poor prognosis. Assessment of the patient's clinical status will often provide the same information. In stable renal failure (such as chronic hemodialysis) or with the use of corticosteroids, prealbumin will be elevated but can still be monitored for trends in the direction of change.

Table 4.3   Factors That Decrease or Increase Prealbumin

Prealbumin	Factors That Decrease Prealbumin	Factors That Increase Prealbumin

Normal: 16–40 mg/dL
Depletion:
  Mild: 10–15 mg/L
  Moderate: 5–9 mg/dL
  Severe: < 5 mg/dL
Half-life approximately 2–3 d
	• Acute-phase response
	• End-stage liver disease (hepatitis, cirrhosis)
	• Untreated hyperthyroidism
	• Nephrotic syndrome
	• Severe zinc deficiency
		• Moderate increase in acute or chronic renal failure
		• Anabolic steroids, possibly glucocorticoids

IMMUNE FUNCTION PARAMETERS

Delayed cutaneous hypersensitivity and reduced total lymphocyte count are two tests that have been used to quantify the impaired immune function associated with uncomplicated malnutrition. However, they are no longer used as part of a routine assessment of hospitalized patients because the inflammatory processes and some therapies, such as chemotherapy and steroids, alter the results (7).

BLOOD GLUCOSE ASSESSMENT

Prediabetes, Type 1 Diabetes Mellitus, and Type 2 Diabetes Mellitus

Diabetes mellitus is a state of chronic hyperglycemia resulting from a deficiency of insulin and/or resistance to the action of insulin. Individuals with type 1 diabetes do not produce appreciable amounts of endogenous insulin and are dependent on exogenous insulin for survival.

Those with type 2 diabetes have either a relative lack of endogenous insulin, impaired insulin receptor function, or both, and can be treated with diet, oral hypoglycemic agents, insulin, or a combination of these three therapies. Although marked hyperglycemia is symptomatic, mild to moderate elevations in blood glucose are often asymptomatic and can go undetected. The American Diabetes Association recommends screening all adults for diabetes or prediabetes (impaired fasting glucose or impaired glucose tolerance) beginning at age 45. If the blood glucose level is normal (70–109 mg/dL), screening should be repeated every 3 years. If the individual has prediabetes, blood glucose levels should be monitored every 1 to 2 years. Consider screening at a younger age or retesting more frequently if the individual has a BMI ≥ 25 and has additional risk factors (eg, is physically inactive, has a first-degree relative with diabetes, is a member of a high-risk ethnic population, has delivered a baby weighing > 9 pounds, has hypertension, has HDL cholesterol < 35 mg/dL or triglycerides > 250 mg/dL, has a condition associated with insulin resistance, or has a history of gestational diabetes or vascular disease) (8).

Diabetes mellitus can be diagnosed using any of the criteria listed in Box 4.2 (9); however, confirmation by repeat testing on a different day is required.

Box 4.2   Criteria for the Diagnosis of Diabetes Mellitus

1. Symptoms of diabetes plus casual plasma glucose concentration ≥ 200 mg/dL (11.1 mmol/L). Casual is defined as any time of day without regard to time since last meal. The classic symptoms of diabetes include polyuria, polydipsia, and unexplained weight loss.

                        OR

2. FPG ≥ 126 mg/dL (7.0 mmol/L). Fasting is defined as no caloric intake for at least 8 h.

                        OR

3. 2-h postload glucose ≥ 200 mg/dL (11.1 mmol/L) during an OGTT. The test should be performed as described by WHO, using a glucose load containing the equivalent of 75 g anhydrous glucose dissolved in water.

In the absence of unequivocal hyperglycemia, these criteria should be confirmed by repeat testing on a different day. The third measure (OGTT) is not recommended for routine clinical use.

Use of intensive insulin therapy to achieve tight glycemic control (80–110 mg/dL) reduces morbidity and mortality in diabetic and nondiabetic critically ill surgical patients compared to conventional treatment to maintain glucose between 180 and 200 mg/dL (10,11). Less dramatic results have been observed in medical ICU patients (12). The American Diabetes Association and American Association of Clinical Endocrinologists (AACE) have developed blood glucose targets for hospitalized patients (13,14) (Table 4.4). Maintaining tight glycemic control increases the occurrence of hypoglycemic events. Due to the risks associated with hypoglycemia, a protocol should be in place to prevent and treat occurrences.

Table 4.4   Blood Glucose Targets for Hospitalized Patients

Patient Acuity	American Diabetes Association	American Association of Clinical Endocrinologists
Noncritically ill	• Premeal as close to 90–130 mg/dL (midpoint of range 110 mg/dL) as possible given the clinical situation • Peak postprandial < 180 mg/dL	• Preprandial < 110 mg/dL • Peak postprandial < 180 mg/dL
Critically ill	• As close to 110 mg/dL as possible and generally < 180 mg/dL	• 80–110 mg/dL

Data are from references 13 and 14.

In patients with diabetes, chronic hyperglycemia is associated with an increased risk of microvascular (retinopathy, nephropathy, and neuropathy) and macrovascular (coronary heart disease and peripheral vascular and cerebrovascular disease) complications. Intensive glycemic control clearly reduces the onset of microvascular and neurologic complications (15). One long-term trial found that tight glycemic control was associated with a reduced risk of cardiovascular complications in type 1 diabetes (16). Nevertheless, large clinical trials are necessary to clarify the extent to which tight glycemic control can prevent or delay macrovascular complications in type 1 and type 2 diabetes (15). The AACE encourages all patients with diabetes to maintain glycemic control as close to normal as possible without causing clinically significant hypoglycemia with goals of fasting glucose < 110 mg/dL and 2-hour postprandial glucose < 140 mg/dL (14).

Gestational Diabetes Mellitus

At the first prenatal visit, risk of gestational diabetes mellitus (GDM) should be assessed. Pregnant women at high risk of GDM (eg, women with marked obesity, a history of GDM, glycosuria, and/or a strong family history) should undergo glucose testing; if results are negative, testing should be repeated between 24 and 28 weeks of gestation. Women with average risk should undergo glucose testing between 24 and 28 weeks of gestation. It may not be cost effective to routinely screen women at low risk for GDM (ie, those meeting *all* the following criteria: < 25 years of age, normal body weight, no family history of diabetes, no previous abnormal glucose tolerance, no history of poor obstetric outcome, not of an ethnic/racial group with a high prevalence of diabetes) (8).

Evaluating Blood Glucose Levels

Abnormalities in blood glucose most commonly occur in type 1 or type 2 diabetes (2,8,17). However, the differential diagnoses include the factors listed in Table 4.5.

Table 4.5   Potential Causes and Symptoms of Hypoglycemia and Hyperglycemia

Hypoglycemia	*Hyperglycemia*
Potential Causes	
• *Treatment of diabetes:* dose of insulin or oral agent is excessive, inappropriately timed, or the wrong type; inadequate glucose (missed meal); increased glucose use (exercise); increased insulin sensitivity (effective intensive therapy); decreased endogenous glucose production (alcohol); decreased insulin clearance (renal failure)	• *Diabetes:* type 1 (autoimmune or idiopathic beta-cell destruction), type 2 (insulin resistance or relative insulin deficiency), gestational (insulin resistance)
• *Medications:* insulin, oral hypoglycemic agents (especially sulfonylureas), alcohol, pentamidine	• *Impaired exocrine pancreas:* pancreatitis, pancreatectomy, pancreatic cancer, hemochromatosis, cystic fibrosis, rare genetic defects
• *Fasting hypoglycemia:* critical illness (severe hepatic or renal disease, sepsis), non-ß-cell tumors, insulinoma	• *Medications:* glucocorticoids, thiazide diuretics,[a] phenytoin, epinephrine
• *Postprandial (reactive) hypoglycemia:* idiopathic, rapid gastric emptying (eg, postgastrectomy), abrupt discontinuation of PN or other rapid dextrose infusions	• *Excess counterregulatory hormones:*[b] trauma, infection, or autonomous endocrine diseases (eg, acromegaly, Cushing's syndrome, pheochromocytoma, glucagonoma, hyperthyroidism)
• *Deficient counterregulatory hormones:*[b] glucagon and/or epinephrine (type 1 DM), rarely cortisol or growth hormone deficiency	• *Excessive dextrose:* high dextrose IV fluid or PN; absorption from high dextrose dialysate fluid
	• *Chromium deficiency* (very rare)
Potential Symptoms	
Sweating, tremor, anxiety, tachycardia, hunger, weakness, dizziness, headache, confusion that may progress to seizures and loss of consciousness	Polyuria, polydipsia, polyphagia, weight loss, fatigue, blurred vision, impaired wound healing, increased susceptibility to infection

[a]Thiazide diuretics include hydrochlorothiazide, chlorthalidone, indapamide, and metolazone.
[b]Glucagon, cortisol, catecholamines (epinephrine and norepinephrine) and growth hormone.

Monitoring Long-Term Glucose Control

The normal range for hemoglobin A_{1c} is approximately 4.0% to 6.0%, using a Diabetes Control and Complications Trial (DCCT)–based assay (8).

Glycated hemoglobin (the A1C test or HbA_{1c}) reflects the patient's mean plasma glucose level during the preceding 2 to 3 months (see Table 4.6) (18). A 1% rise in the A1C test represents approximately a 35-mg/dL increase in the mean plasma glucose (8).

Table 4.6   Approximate Mean Plasma Glucose Corresponding with Glycated Hemoglobin (AIC Test) Results

Glycated Hemoglobin (A1C), %	Mean Plasma Glucose, mg/dL[a]
6	135
7	170
8	205
9	240
10	275
11	310
12	345

[a]On multiple testing over 2–3 months.

Copyright © 2007 American Diabetes Association. From Diabetes Care®, Vol. 30, 2007; S4-S41. Modified with permission from the American Diabetes Association.

A baseline A1C test measurement should be evaluated upon diagnosis of diabetes mellitus. Frequency of monitoring the A1C test will depend on the treatment regimen and judgment of the clinician. It is recommended that the test be given at least 2 times a year if glycemic control is adequate, and every 3 months to patients whose therapy has changed or who demonstrate poor control. The American Diabetes Association A1C goal for patients in general is < 7% and for the individual patient is as close to < 6% (normal) as feasible without hypoglycemia (8). A1C goals for children and adolescents are higher (7% to 8%) because of the risk for impairment of cognitive function by frequent hypoglycemic events (8).

The A1C test reflects the amount of glucose bound to hemoglobin over the red blood cells' (RBC) life span. Consequently, results are falsely low in diseases that shorten RBC lifespan (eg, sickle cell, hemolytic anemias, and chronic blood loss) and are falsely high after a splenectomy (2).

Diabetic Ketoacidosis and Hyperosmolar, Hyperglycemic State

Insulin deficiency, increased counterregulatory hormones, and volume depletion can result in diabetic ketoacidosis (DKA) or hyperosmolar hyperglycemic state (HHS), occurring most frequently in type 1 and type 2 diabetes, respectively (19). See Table 4.7 (20).

Table 4.7   Laboratory Abnormalities Often Seen with Diabetic Ketoacidosis and Hyperosmolar, Hyperglycemic State

Laboratory Abnormalities	Diabetic Ketoacidosis (Mild to Severe)	Hyperosmolar Hyperglycemic State
Hyperglycemia	Plasma glucose > 250 mg/dL	Plasma glucose > 600 mg/dL
Ketosis:[a] ketones in urine and/or blood	Positive	Small
Metabolic acidosis	Arterial pH < 7.0–7.3 Serum bicarbonate < 10–18 mEq/L Anion gap >10–12	pH > 7.3 Serum bicarbonate > 15 mEq/L Anion gap variable
Electrolyte shifts	Despite a total-body deficit, serum potassium is initially normal to elevated, then drops rapidly with correction of the acidosis, insulin therapy, and volume expansion	Normal serum potassium
Serum osmolality	Variable	> 320 mOsm/kg water

[a]Nitroprusside reaction method. Ketosis is also seen in alcoholism, starvation, very-low-carbohydrate diets, and up to 30% of first-morning urine samples during pregnancy.

Copyright © 2004 American Diabetes Association. From *Diabetes Care*®, Vol. 27, 2004; S94-S102. Modified with permission from the American Diabetes Association.

ELECTROLYTE ASSESSMENT

Sodium: Hyponatremia
(serum sodium < 135 mEq/L) (2,17,21–25)

Hypo- and hypernatremia are disorders of sodium concentration in the serum, not of total-body sodium. Serum sodium concentrations correlate poorly with the need for sodium repletion and are typically more reflective of total-body water than sodium balance. Evaluation of abnormal serum sodium concentrations requires a simultaneous examination of volume status to determine the cause and appropriate therapy. Hyponatremia can be present with decreased, normal, or increased total-body water and/or sodium. True sodium depletion (decreased total-body sodium) is uncommon. However, it can occur as a result of the replacement of gastrointestinal (GI) or renal losses with free water or other hypotonic fluids (eg, D_5W, ¼ NS, or ½ NS).

Symptoms are uncommon unless serum sodium declines rapidly or falls below ~ 120–125 mEq/L, at which point nausea, vomiting, headache, lethargy, and mental-status changes (eg, confusion or psychosis) can occur. In cases of severe hyponatremia (~ < 115 mEq/L), convulsions, seizures, coma, and even death may occur. The correction of hyponatremia should proceed at a gradual rate, because aggressive treatment can precipitate neurologic sequelae (central pontine myelinolysis).

An important step in diagnostic evaluation of hyponatremia is to measure or calculate serum osmolality.

Calculated serum osmolality = (2 × serum Na) + (serum glucose/18) + (serum BUN/2.8)

Where: BUN = blood urea nitrogen in mg/dL; Na = sodium in mEq/L.

When hyponatremia is associated with decreased serum osmolality (< 280 mOsm/kg H_2O), it is essential to simultaneously evaluate the patient's volume status (ie, extracellular fluid volume [ECF]). As indicated in Table 4.8 (22,24,25), this will help determine the etiology and appropriate treatment (see also the Hydration Status section of this chapter and Chapter 3, Nutrition-Focused Physical Assessment). Table 4.9 outlines the etiologies and treatment when hyponatremia is associated with an increased or normal serum osmolality, which are less common manifestations of hyponatremia.

Table 4.8 Evaluation of Hyponatremia When Serum Osmolality Is Low (< 280 mOsm/kg H_2O)

Extracellular Fluid Volume (ECF) Finding	Signs/Symptoms	Possible Causes	Treatment
Volume depletion (hypovolemic hypotonic hyponatremia): total-body water deficit with larger total-body sodium deficit	• Tachycardia, low blood pressure, decreased skin turgor • Urine Na^+ < 20 mEq/L usually indicates extrarenal losses • Urine Na^+ > 20 mEq/L usually indicates renal losses	*Extrarenal losses* • Gastrointestinal tract: diarrhea (especially secretory), vomiting, gastric suction, fistula • Skin: burns, excessive sweating • Third spacing: ascites, bowel obstruction, peritonitis, pancreatitis • Lungs: bronchorrhea *Renal losses* • Diuretics • Renal disease: renal tubular acidosis, salt-wasting nephropathy • Osmotic diuresis: ketones, glucose, urea • Primary adrenal insufficiency Treat underlying cause. Volume	expansion; replete with isotonic fluids (eg, NS or lactated Ringer's). Replace ongoing losses with fluids containing a similar composition.

(continues next page)

Table 4.8 Evaluation of Hyponatremia When Serum Osmolality Is Low (< 280 mOsm/kg H$_2$O) (continued)

Extracellular Fluid Volume (ECF) Finding	Signs/Symptoms	Possible Causes	Treatment
Euvolemic or modest ECF volume excess (isovolemic hypotonic hyponatremia): normal to moderately increased total-body water ± total-body sodium	• Normal pulse, blood pressure and skin turgor; no edema • Urine Na$^+$ usually > 20 mEq/L	• SIADH • Glucocorticoid deficiency • Hypothyroidism • Polydipsia • Reset osmostat syndrome (cachexia, malnutrition) • Iatrogenic (eg, renal failure with provision of hypotonic fluid exceeding excretory capacity) • Potassium depletion	Treat underlying cause. Water restriction.
Volume expansion (hypervolemic hypotonic hyponatremia): excess total-body sodium with larger excess of total-body water	• Edema • Urine Na$^+$ < 20 mEq/L usually indicates edema-forming states • Urine Na$^+$ > 20 mEq/L usually indicates renal failure	• Edema-forming states: congestive heart failure, cirrhosis, nephrotic syndrome • Acute or chronic renal failure	Treat underlying cause. Sodium and water restriction.

Adapted from: Avner ED. Clinical disorders of water metabolism: hyponatremia and hypernatremia. *Pediatr Ann.* 1995;24:23–30; Whitmire SJ. Fluids, electrolytes and acid-base balance. In: Matarese LM, Gottschlich MM, eds. *Contemporary Nutrition Support Practice: A Clinical Guide.* 2nd ed. Philadelphia, PA: WB Saunders; 2003:130; and Narins RG, Jones ER, Stom MC, Rudnick MR, Bastl CP. Diagnostic strategies in disorders of fluid, electrolyte and acid-base homeostasis. *Am J Med.* 1982;72:496–520. Whitmire and Narins are adapted with permission from Elsevier.

Table 4.9   Evaluation of Hyponatremia When Serum Osmolality Is Normal (280–295 mOsm/kg H₂O) or High (> 295 mOsm/kg H₂O)

	Normal Serum Osmolality (Iso-osmolar Hyponatremia)	*High Serum Osmolality (Hyperosmolar Hyponatremia)*
Possible causes	• Infusion of isotonic, sodium-free solutions (eg, during transurethral resection of the prostate or bladder) • Pseudohyponatremia[b]	• Hyperglycemia[a] • Infusion of hypertonic, sodium-free solutions (eg, mannitol) • Toxins
Treatment	Treat underlying cause	Treat underlying cause

[a]Serum sodium is falsely decreased by approximately 1.6 mEq/L for each 100 mg/dL rise in glucose. The adjustment in serum sodium should be calculated in hyperglycemic conditions.
[b]Pseudohyponatremia is an artifactually low sodium concentration that can occur (with hyperlipidemia or hyperproteinemia) if using the flame photometric laboratory techniques and does not warrant treatment to correct hyponatremia.

Adapted from: Avner ED. Clinical disorders of water metabolism: hyponatremia and hypernatremia. *Pediatr Ann.* 1995;24:23–30; Whitmire SJ. Fluids, electrolytes and acid-base balance. In: Matarese LM, Gottschlich MM, eds. *Contemporary Nutrition Support Practice: A Clinical Guide.* 2nd ed. Philadelphia, PA: WB Saunders; 2003:130; and Narins RG, Jones ER, Stom MC, Rudnick MR, Bastl CP. Diagnostic strategies in disorders of fluid, electrolyte and acid-base homeostasis. *Am J Med.* 1982;72:496–520. Whitmire and Narins are adapted with permission from Elsevier.

Sodium: Hypernatremia (serum sodium > 145 mEq/L) (2,17,21–25)

Hypernatremia is much less common than hyponatremia but is associated with a high morbidity and mortality. Sodium is the main cation in ECF and, along with accompanying anions, is the primary determinant of serum osmolality. Serum osmolality is not useful to evaluate the etiology of hypernatremia because it is always elevated in hypernatremic states. However, it can be useful to monitor the severity and progress of correction. As hypernatremia reflects a derangement of the relative amounts of sodium and water, an evaluation of hypernatremia must be done in conjunction with an assessment of volume status to identify the etiology and appropriate treatment strategy. Most commonly, hypernatremia is associated with a water deficit (dehydration) and is rarely due to a gain in total-body sodium. An estimation of free-water deficit can be calculated using serum sodium levels:

Free-water deficit in liters =
$(1 - [140/\text{serum Na mEq}]) \times (0.6 \times \text{body weight in kg})$

Hypernatremia essentially never occurs in a patient with a normal thirst mechanism and access to water. The elderly are at risk of dehydration because of declining renal sodium conservation and diminished thirst perception.

The onset of symptoms will depend on both the rate and degree of increased serum sodium. Early signs include thirst and dry mucous membranes. Neurologic signs, such as drowsiness, lethargy, disorientation, and confusion, are observed as water progressively shifts from intracellular fluid (ICF) spaces into the hyperosmolar ECF. Severe hypernatremia can result in respiratory paralysis, coma, and ultimately, death. Refer to Table 4.10 (24,25) for information regarding the evaluation of ECF and hypernatremia. See also the Hydration Status section of this chapter and Chapter 3, Nutrition-Focused Physical Assessment.

Table 4.10 Hypernatremia and Evaluation of Extracellular Fluid (ECF) Volume

ECF Finding	Urine Na⁺	Possible Causes	Treatment
Volume depletion (hypovolemic hypernatremia): total-body sodium deficit with larger total-body water deficit	< 20 mEq/L indicates extrarenal losses > 20 mEq/L indicates renal losses	*Extrarenal losses* • Gastrointestinal tract: severe diarrhea (especially osmotic), vomiting, fistula losses • Skin: excessive sweating, burns • Lungs: bronchorrhea, hyperventilation *Renal losses* • Diuresis: diuretics, osmotic diuresis (glucosuria, diuretic phase of acute tubular necrosis) • Partial urinary tract obstruction • Renal dysplasia	Volume expansion: initially use isotonic fluids (eg, NS, lactated Ringer's). After hemodynamic stability and good urine output, change to hypotonic saline.
Euvolemia or modest ECF volume loss (isovolemic hypernatremia): total-body water loss with normal total-body sodium	Variable	*Extrarenal losses* • Skin losses: especially if replacement is NS • Lung losses: hyperventilation • Water deprivation: inadequate access to water, hypodypsia *Renal losses*	*Renal losses* Treat underlying cause; water replacement

(continues next page)

Table 4.10 Hypernatremia and Evaluation of Extracellular Fluid (ECF) Volume (continued)

ECF Finding	Urine Na$^+$	Possible Causes	Treatment
		• Renal losses	
		• Diabetes insipidus (central or nephrogenic)	
Volume expansion[a] (hypervolemic hypernatremia): total-body sodium excess greater than total-body water excess (uncommon)	> 20 mEq/L	• Iatrogenic sodium administration: inappropriate use of NaCl, NaHCO$_3$, hypertonic dialysis, high-sodium medications (salt tablets, sodium-salt antibiotics), or, rarely, excess dietary sodium • Mineralocorticoid excess: hyperaldosteronism, Cushing's disease, congenital adrenal hyperplasia	Decrease sodium in intravenous fluids, PN, and medications. Remove sodium with diuretics (or dialysis, if in renal failure); water replacement.

[a] In hypervolemic hypernatremia, overt evidence of ECF volume expansion may not be evident on physical examination.

Adapted from: Avner ED. Clinical disorders of water metabolism: hyponatremia and hypernatremia. *Pediatr Ann.* 1995;24:23–30; and Whitmire SJ. Fluids, electrolytes and acid-base balance. In: Matarese LM, Gottschlich MM, eds. *Contemporary Nutrition Support Practice: A Clinical Guide.* 2nd ed. Philadelphia, PA: WB Saunders; 2003:132. Whitmire adapted with permission from Elsevier.

Potassium
(normal serum: 3.5–5.0 mEq/L) (2,17,21,23,24)

Potassium is the major intracellular fluid (ICF) cation, with less than 2% of total-body stores in ECF. Serum levels do not correlate well with body stores. However, in the absence of acid-base disturbances or transcellular shifts, a low serum potassium level may provide a rough estimation of the depleted body stores. A decline in serum potassium from 4.0 to 3.0 mEq/L may correlate with an estimated deficit of 200–400 mEq; a level < 3.0 mEq/L may require > 600 mEq to replete body potassium stores. Frequent monitoring is required to assess the response during repletion. With refractory hypokalemia, serum magnesium should also be monitored, as potassium repletion is impaired in magnesium-deficient states.

Chronic hyperkalemia is usually due to impaired renal excretion. A spurious elevation in serum potassium is possible if the blood sample is hemolyzed during phlebotomy or if it contains very high platelets (thrombocytosis) or white blood cells (leukocytosis). Serum potassium can also be falsely elevated if the blood is drawn from a vein or inadequately flushed IV line into which potassium is being infused (eg, PN). If the blood sample is contaminated with PN, the glucose will typically also be elevated. A repeat blood sample should be obtained. Serum potassium is increased by approximately 0.6 mEq/L for each 0.1-drop in pH, or decreased 0.6 with each 0.1-increase in pH. Correction of an acid-base disturbance will adjust the serum potassium level.

**Box 4.3   Factors That Decrease Serum Potassium and
            Signs/Symptoms of Hypokalemia**

Factors That Can Cause Hypokalemia

- *Renal losses:* osmotic diuresis, hypomagnesemia, hyperaldosteronism, Cushing's syndrome, or Bartter's syndrome, licorice excess
- *GI losses:* diarrhea, intestinal or biliary fistula, ureterosigmoidostomy, villous adenoma, prolonged vomiting or gastric suction
- *Medications:* loop[a] or thiazide[b] diuretics, amphotericin B, cisplatin, insulin, Beta $_2$ adrenergic agonists,[c] foscarnet, high-dose glucocorticoids or penicillins
- *Shift into cells:* alkalosis, anabolism, refeeding syndrome, correction of hyperglycemia or diabetic ketoacidosis (DKA)
- *Inadequate intake (seldom the sole cause):* anorexia nervosa, malnutrition, alcoholism, intravenous hydration without potassium

Signs and Symptoms of Hypokalemia

- ~ < 3.0 mEq/L: muscle weakness, myalgias, constipation, ileus, decreased deep-tendon reflexes
- EKG changes: flat or inverted T wave, increased U wave, depressed ST segment, arrhythmias

---

[a]Loop diuretics include furosemide, bumetanide, ethacrynic acid, torsemide.
[b]Thiazide diuretics include hydrochlorothiazide.
[c]Beta $_2$ adrenergic agonists include isoproterenol, epinephrine, terbutaline.

Box 4.4   Factors That Increase Serum Potassium and Signs/Symptoms of Hyperkalemia

---

Factors That Can Cause Hyperkalemia
- *Decreased renal excretion:* acute oliguric renal failure, chronic renal failure, hypoaldosteronism, type IV renal tubular acidosis
- *Medications:* potassium sparing diuretics,[a] beta blockers,[b] angiotensin-converting enzyme (ACE) inhibitors,[c] cyclosporine, heparin, digitalis toxicity, trimethoprim, tacrolimus, pentamidine, non-steroidal anti-inflammatory drugs (NSAIDs)
- *Shift out of cells:* acidosis, massive cellular destruction (tissue necrosis, rhabdomyolysis, GI hemorrhage, hemolysis, hemolytic anemia)

Signs and Symptoms of Hyperkalemia
- Muscle weakness, paresthesias, decreased deep-tendon reflexes, flaccid paralysis
- ~ > 7.0 potentially life threatening. EKG changes: peaked T waves; prolonged PR interval, wide QRS, small or absent P waves, ventricular arrhythmias. Finally, QRS degenerates into a sine wave and cardiac arrest

---

[a]Potassium-sparing diuretics include amiloride, triamterene, spironolactone.
[b]Beta blockers include propranolol, metoprolol, atenolol; they rarely cause hyperkalemia alone but contribute to elevations with other conditions.
[c]ACE inhibitors include captopril, enalapril, quinapril, ramipril.

Calcium (normal serum 9.0–10.5 mg/dL, normal ionized 4.5–5.6 mg/dL) (2,17,21,23,24)

Less than 1% of the body's calcium is present in ECF. Normal serum calcium levels are primarily maintained by hormonal regulation (parathyroid hormone, vitamin D, and calcitonin). Large skeletal reserves help to compensate for inadequate calcium intake or reduced GI absorption (seen with a diet high in phosphorus, oxalate, or phytate). Total serum calcium reflects the ionized calcium, plus calcium bound to protein (primarily albumin) and anions. The equations to adjust serum calcium for hypoalbuminemia are not reliable for use in acute care because of poor sensitivity and a high rate of false negatives (26). Ionized calcium is a more accurate reflection of the physiologically active calcium level and should be evaluated before initiating calcium repletion, especially in patients with hypoalbuminemia. Furthermore, serum magnesium and phosphorus levels should also be measured and, if low, treated in patients with hypocalcemia.

Typically, hypercalcemia occurs when excessive calcium from the intestine and/or bone enters the ECF and exceeds the renal excretory capacity. A high calcium intake may increase serum calcium to 0.5 mg/dL (see Box 4.6).

Box 4.5   Factors That Decrease Serum Calcium and Signs/Symptoms of Hypocalcemia

Factors That Can Cause Hypocalcemia
- Hypoalbuminemia[a]
- Hypoparathyroidism
- Hypomagnesemia
- Renal failure, renal tubular acidosis
- Vitamin D deficiency or impaired metabolism
- Medications: foscarnet, loop diuretics,[b] anticonvulsants,[c] cisplatin, plicamycin, gentamicin, corticosteroids, calcitonin, colchicine
- Hyperphosphatemia
- Acute pancreatitis
- Hungry bone syndrome[d]
- Citrated blood products

Signs and Symptoms of Hypocalcemia
- Often asymptomatic; symptoms reflect degree and acuteness of decline in serum
- Paresthesias of fingers/toes/mouth, muscle cramps, nonspecific psychiatric changes
- Severe ~< 2.0 mg/dL ionized calcium: positive Chvostek's[e] or Trousseau's sign,[f] tetany, muscle spasms, hyperactive reflexes, EKG changes: prolonged QT and ST intervals, convulsions, seizures, refractory hypotension, arrhythmias, bradycardia, cardiac arrest
- Chronic: dry/scaly skin, brittle nails, coarse hair, cataracts

[a]The total serum calcium level will be decreased by hypoalbuminemia; however, the ionized calcium will be unchanged. Obtain an ionized calcium level or calculate the corrected calcium:
Corrected calcium = total serum calcium mg/dL + 0.8 (4.0 — serum albumin g/dL)
[b]Loop diuretics include furosemide, bumetanide, ethacrynic acid.
[c]Anticonvulsants include phenobarbital, phenytoin, carbamazepine, primidone.
[d]Hungry bone syndrome occurs in some patients after a parathyroidectomy and is characterized by rapid/excessive osteogenesis that can result in hypocalcemia.
[e]Chvostek's sign: A twitch of the facial muscles upon tapping the facial nerve in front of the ear.
[f]Trousseau's sign: A hand spasm observed when the blood pressure cuff is inflated to above systolic blood pressure for up to 3 minutes.

Box 4.6   Factors That Increase Serum Calcium and Signs/Symptoms of Hypercalcemia

Factors That Can Cause Hypercalcemia
- Hyperparathyroidism
- Some malignancies (with or without metastasis to the bone), especially breast, lung, or kidney; multiple myeloma, leukemia, or lymphoma
- Medications: thiazide diuretics,[a] lithium, vitamin A toxicity
- Immobilization
- Hyperthyroidism
- Less common: excess 1,25-dihydroxyvitamin D, tuberculosis, sarcoidosis, milk-alkali syndrome, after renal transplantation, diuretic phase of acute renal failure

Signs and Symptoms of Hypercalcemia
- Mild: often asymptomatic; typically nonspecific
- Symptomatic ~> 11.5 mg/dL total calcium: nausea, vomiting, anorexia, polydipsia, polyuria, dehydration, muscle weakness, fatigability, hyporeflexia, constipation, mental changes, confusion, depression, EKG changes: shortened QT interval, bradyarrhythmias ~> 18 mg/dL may cause shock, renal failure, coma, death
- Chronic: with increased phosphorus can cause soft-tissue deposits,[b] hypertension

[a]Thiazide diuretics include hydrochlorothiazide.
[b]The calcium-phosphorus product (ie, [serum calcium in mg/dL] × [serum phosphorus in mg/dL]) should not be > 70 mg/dL.

Phosphorus
(normal serum 3.0–4.5 mg/dL) (2,17,21,23,24)

Phosphorus is the primary intracellular anion. The serum phosphorus level is a poor reflection of body stores, because < 1% is present in ECF, and the bones serve as a reservoir that can buffer changes in serum or intracellular phosphorus. However, recommendations for empiric replacement based on serum levels can be used as a rough guide. Oral or enteral supplementation is the preferred route; however, intravenous replacement therapy is usually warranted in profound hypophosphatemia (< 1.0 mg/dL) if the patient is symptomatic or when oral replacement therapy is limited by GI side effects. Response to supplementation is unpredictable and should be monitored closely.

Hyperphosphatemia is most commonly due to impaired renal excretion. Serum phosphorus can be artifactually elevated by hemolysis of the blood sample; thrombocytosis and multiple myeloma can also cause spurious elevations.

Box 4.7   Factors That Decrease Serum Phosphorus and Signs/Symptoms of Hypophosphatemia

---

Factors That Can Cause Hypophosphatemia
- *Impaired absorption:* malabsorption, diarrhea, vitamin D deficiency or impaired metabolism
- *Medications:* phosphate binding antacids,[a] sucralfate, steroids (anabolic and glucocorticoid), insulin, epinephrine
- Alcoholism
- *Intracellular shifts:* alkalosis (especially respiratory), cellular uptake (anabolism, some neoplasms), burn (especially recovery), sepsis
- Refeeding syndrome
- *Increased losses:* hyperparathyroidism, renal tubular defects (Fanconi syndrome), DKA (the recovery phase), hypomagnesemia, diuretic phase of ATN (briefly) or after renal transplantation
- *Inadequate intake:* PN or dextrose-based IVF without adequate phosphorus

Signs and Symptoms of Hypophosphatemia
- Mild: usually asymptomatic
- Severe (< 1.0–1.5 mg/dL): anorexia, confusion, irritability, muscle weakness, paresthesias, decreased diaphragmatic contractility, ataxia, seizure, RBC dysfunction, thrombocytopenia, hemolysis, rhabdomyolysis, coma, respiratory failure/arrest

---

[a]Phosphate-binding antacids include those that are aluminum based (aluminum hydroxide) and those that are calcium based (calcium acetate, carbonate, or gluconate).

**Box 4.8   Factors That Increase Serum Phosphorus and
Signs/Symptoms of Hyperphosphatemia**

Factors That Can Cause Hyperphosphatemia
- *Decreased renal excretion:* acute or chronic renal failure,
  hypoparathyroidism, acromegaly
- *Increased cellular release:* tumor lysis syndrome, tissue
  necrosis, rhabdomyolysis
- *Increased exogenous phosphorus load or absorption:*
  phosphorus-containing laxatives or enemas, vitamin D excess
- Acidosis (shift into ECF)

Signs and Symptoms of Hyperphosphatemia
- Usually asymptomatic
- Hypocalcemia
- Chronic: if calcium phosphorus product remains > 70 mg/dL,
  can see soft-tissue deposits or joint calcification

Magnesium
(normal serum 1.3–2.1 mEq/L) (2,17,21,23,24)

Serum levels may not accurately reflect body stores,
because only about 1% of magnesium is present in ECF.
Hypomagnesemia is usually due to inadequate intake in
conjunction with increased renal losses or impaired GI
absorption. Magnesium depletion is commonly seen in
critically ill patients, alcoholics, and in diabetic patients
with osmotic diuresis. Hypocalcemia and hypokalemia are
frequently associated with hypomagnesemia and are
refractory to repletion until the magnesium deficit is corrected. Clinical manifestations of hypomagnesemia are
similar to hypocalcemia and can be exacerbated if both are
present. Oral magnesium replacement can result in diarrhea. Intravenous or intramuscular repletion is recommended for severe and/or symptomatic cases.

Normal kidneys can excrete excess magnesium efficiently; therefore, chronic hypermagnesemia is usually associated with renal failure. Symptomatic hypermagnesemia is fairly uncommon.

Box 4.9 Factors That Decrease Serum Magnesium and Signs/Symptoms of Hypomagnesemia

---

Factors That Can Cause Hypomagnesemia

- *Decreased absorption:* prolonged diarrhea, intestinal or biliary fistula, intestinal resection or bypass, steatorrhea, ulcerative colitis; to a lesser extent upper GI fluid losses: prolonged gastric suction, excessive vomiting
- *Renal losses:* osmotic diuresis, DM/glucosuria, correction of DKA, renal disease with magnesium wasting, hypophosphatemia, hypercalcemia, hyperthyroidism, hyperaldosteronism, diuretic phase of acute tubular necrosis, renal tubular acidosis, inherited renal tubular defects
- Alcoholism
- *Inadequate intake:* malnutrition
- *Medications:* diuretics,[a] amphotericin B, aminoglycosides,[b] cisplatin, cyclosporine, pentamidine, foscarnet, tacrolimus
- *Intracellular shift:* acute pancreatitis
- Refeeding syndrome

Signs and Symptoms of Hypomagnesemia

- ~ < 0.5–1.0 mEq/L: muscle weakness, anorexia, nausea, mental status changes (confusion, depression, psychosis), hypocalcemia with positive Chvostek's[c] or, less frequently, Trousseau's sign,[d] muscle tremors progressing to seizures, tetany
- Flat or inverted T wave (a sign of either hypomagnesemia or hypokalemia); increased PT and QT interval; ventricular arrhythmias

---

[a] Mild hypomagnesemia can occur with loop or thiazide diuretics.
[b] Aminoglycoside antibiotics include gentamicin and tobramycin.
[c] Chvostek's sign: A twitch of the facial muscles upon tapping the facial nerve in front of the ear.
[d] Trousseau's sign: A hand spasm observed when the blood pressure cuff is inflated to above systolic blood pressure for up to 3 minutes.

**Box 4.10   Factors That Increase Serum Magnesium[a] and
Signs/Symptoms of Hypermagnesemia**

Factors That Can Cause Hypermagnesemia
• Acute or chronic renal failure

The following seldom cause significant/chronic
hypermagnesemia unless renal function is also impaired:
• *Medications:* magnesium-rich cathartics and antacids,[b]
  administration of magnesium to suppress premature labor
• Rhabdomyolysi*s*
• Adrenal insufficiency (Addison's disease)
• Hypothyroidism
• Dehydration

Signs and Symptoms of Hypermagnesemia
• Diminished deep-tendon reflexes, EKG changes: prolonged
  PR interval; also peaked T wave, wide QRS complex (can be
  either hypermagnesemia or hyperkalemia), arrhythmias,
  mental confusion
• Respiratory depression, respiratory muscle paralysis,
  peripheral vasodilation resulting in profound hypotension
• ~> 12–15 mEq/L can cause cardiac arrest

---

[a]Note that laboratory error may lead to incorrect serum magnesium results.
Artifactual increases are seen with hemolysis or decreases with hypoalbuminemia.
[b]Magnesium-rich cathartics include magnesium citrate and milk of magnesia.
Magnesium-containing antacids include Maalox and Mylanta.

ACID-BASE ASSESSMENT

Acid-Base Disorders (2,21,22,24,27)

The pH is a measure of acidity/alkalinity based on the
number of hydrogen ions (H^+) present. Acids by definition
are H^+ donors, such as hydrochloric acid; bases are H^+
acceptors, including bicarbonate, acetate, citrate, lactate,
and gluconate. The arterial pH is maintained within a nar-
row physiologic range (7.35–7.45) by the combined action

of the lungs, via control of the partial pressure of carbon dioxide in the blood (PCO_2), and of the kidneys via control of bicarbonate and acid excretion and the production of buffers. Some nonrenal buffer systems also exist.

Metabolic acid-base disorders manifest as changes in serum chloride and bicarbonate (HCO_3), whereas respiratory acid-base disorders are characterized by abnormalities in PCO_2. The body attempts to compensate for a primary *metabolic* acid-base disorder with "secondary" or "compensatory" *respiratory* changes. The lungs usually respond within minutes to compensate by adjusting minute ventilation (ie, respiratory rate x tidal volume), in order to retain or release carbon dioxide. Large amounts of acid can be removed when hydrogen ions (H^+) are buffered by bicarbonate and converted to water and CO_2, which is expired by the lungs. Conversely, hypoventilation can help to conserve acid. A primary *respiratory* acid-base disorder typically elicits a compensatory *renal* response.

The kidneys retain or excrete acid (H^+) and/or base equivalents to maintain serum pH. Metabolic compensation occurs during several hours to days, even in the healthy kidney. Buffers present in body fluids, such as bicarbonate, hemoglobin, proteins, ammonium, and phosphates, can act immediately to help maintain a normal pH.

To evaluate an acid-base disturbance, the pH and PCO_2 are obtained from an arterial blood gas (ABG) sample, along with measurement of serum CO_2 (which consists primarily of HCO_3), sodium, and chloride. Serial measurements are collected and interpreted in conjunction with the patient's clinical status and, if mechanically ventilated, the ventilatory parameters.

Remember to treat the primary disorder—not the compensatory mechanism. If the expected compensation does not occur, it may indicate a second primary disorder (mixed acid-base disorder). However, mixed acid-base disorders are beyond the scope of this handbook. Some metabolic acid-base imbalances may respond to adjustments in acetate and/or chloride content of parenteral nutrition and other IV fluids. Respiratory imbalances will not. However, if a primary respiratory acidosis cannot be corrected by supporting lung function, metabolic compensation may be augmented by adjusting the acetate load of the PN. The composition of enteral feeding will not alter acid-base disturbances. However, if MCT oil is provided in excess of oxidative capacity, increased ketone bodies are produced, which may worsen acidosis.

Overfeeding results in excess CO_2 production. If this exacerbates an acute respiratory acidosis, calories should be limited to maintenance requirements.

Box 4.11   Expected Compensation, Causes, and Treatment of Metabolic Acidosis

Uncompensated:
- pH low (< 7.35)
- HCO_3— low < 21 mEq/L)
- PCO_2 normal (35–45 mm Hg)

Compensated:
- pH near normal
- HCO_3— low
- PCO_2 low
- Respiratory compensation occurs by increasing respiratory rate and/or depth (hyperventilation). PCO_2 should fall approximately 1.3 mm Hg for each 1.0-mEq/L drop in HCO_3—.

Principal Causes:

1. Increased anion gap acidosis* (normochloremic metabolic acidosis)
- Ketoacidosis: diabetic, alcoholic, starvation
- Lactic acidosis: hypoperfusion, shock, severe liver failure, thiamin deficiency
- Acute or chronic renal failure
- Toxic acid ingestion: ethylene glycol, methanol, paraldehyde, salicylate overdose

2. Normal anion gap acidosis[a] (hyperchloremic metabolic acidosis)
- GI HCO_3^- loss: diarrhea, small bowel/biliary/pancreatic drainage or fistula, ureterosigmoidostomy
- Renal HCO_3^- loss, impaired reabsorption, or impaired H^+ excretion: renal tubular acidosis, interstitial nephritis, hypoaldosteronism, early renal insufficiency, obstructive nephropathy
- Iatrogenic: carbonic anhydrase inhibitors (acetazolamide), excess chloride from normal saline, PN, or acidifying agents (ammonium chloride, hydrochloric acid)

(continues next page)

Box 4.11   Expected Compensation, Causes, and Treatment of Metabolic Acidosis (continued)

Treatment:
- Correct underlying defect.
- Supplementation with alkali (eg, sodium bicarbonate[b]) or bicarbonate precursors (eg, sodium citrate) may be appropriate in some cases.
- In PN, increase acetate if significant and/or chronic HCO_3— losses.[b] Decrease chloride if due to excess.
- Hyperkalemia usually resolves with correction of acidosis.

[a]The anion gap is based on the concept that there is a normal difference between the primary measured cation (Na^+) and anions (Cl^-, HCO_3^-). This difference or "gap" helps to determine the etiology of metabolic acidosis, because it is increased when other unmeasured anions are present. Anion gap = (Na^+) — (Cl^- + HCO_3^-). A normal anion gap is 8–12 mEq/L, although it can vary significantly with different laboratories.
[b]Bicarbonate is unstable in PN and is not added because of the risk of precipitation. Acetate and/or lactate are used as bicarbonate precursors that are converted to bicarbonate in the liver.

Box 4.12   Expected Compensation, Causes, and Treatment of Metabolic Alkalosis

Uncompensated:
- pH high (> 7.45)
- HCO_3— high (> 24 mEq/L)
- PCO_2 normal (35–45 mm Hg)

Compensated:
- pH near normal
- HCO_3—high
- PCO_2 high
- Respiration is depressed (hypoventilation) as a compensatory response by the lungs. PCO_2 typically rises about 0.7 mm Hg for each 1.0-mEq/L increase in HCO_3^-.

(continues next page)

Box 4.12   Expected Compensation, Causes, and Treatment of Metabolic Alkalosis (continued)

Principal Causes:

1. Chloride responsive*
- GI loss of chloride and/or acid: gastric drainage, vomiting, laxative abuse, colonic villous adenoma
- Diuretics; volume contraction
- Correction of chronic hypercapnia

2. Chloride unresponsive[a]
- Excess mineralocorticoid: Cushing's syndrome, primary hyperaldosteronism, glucocorticoids, glycyrrhizic acid (licorice), Bartter's syndrome

3. Other
- Excess alkali intake: citrate (Shol's solution, massive blood transfusions, regional citrate anticoagulation during continuous renal replacement therapy. HCO_3^- ($NaHCO_3$, Ringer's lactate, acetate), excessive antacids, PN with excess acetate
- Intracellular H^+ shift: severe potassium depletion

Treatment:
- Correct underlying defect. Replete deficit of chloride, potassium, magnesium, and/or volume. If possible, stop gastric suction, diuretics, and/or excess bicarbonate.
- In PN, increased chloride can be appropriate in the chloride-responsive categories listed above or decreased acetate when excess alkali is the cause.
- Monitor for hypokalemia from renal tubule losses plus a shift from ECF to ICF.

---

[a]Evaluation of urine chloride is sometimes used to aid in diagnosis. A low-urine chloride (< 10 mmol/L) is found in chloride-responsive alkalosis and a high-urine chloride (> 20 mmol/L) is consistent with chloride-unresponsive alkalosis.

Box 4.13   Expected Compensation, Causes, and Treatment of Respiratory Acidosis

---

Uncompensated or Acute < 24 Hours:
- pH low (< 7.35)
- PCO_2 high (> 45 mm Hg = hypercapnia)
- HCO_3^- normal or slightly increased (≥ 21–28 mEq/L)

Compensated or Chronic:
- pH near normal
- PCO_2 high
- HCO_3^-— high
- Renal compensation occurs by the excretion of chloride and retaining HCO_3^-; HCO_3^- rises approximately 3–4 mEq/L for each 10-mm Hg increase in PCO_2.

Principal Causes:
(Hypoventilation with inadequate excretion of CO_2)
- Respiratory center depression: anesthesia, brain injury or tumor, drug overdose (sedative, barbiturate), Pickwickian syndrome, primary hypoventilation
- Restrictive defects: flail chest, hemo- or pneumothorax, pneumonia, kyphoscoliosis, obesity
- Neuromuscular abnormalities: brain stem injury, myasthenia gravis, Guillain-Barré syndrome, multiple sclerosis, muscular dystrophy, amyotrophic lateral sclerosis, diaphragmatic paralysis
- Airway obstruction: aspiration, bronchospasm, sleep apnea, obstructive lung disease (bronchitis, emphysema)
- Respiratory/circulatory collapse: cardiac arrest, severe pulmonary edema, pulmonary embolism

Treatment:
- Correct underlying disturbance.
- Supplement oxygen or mechanical ventilation as needed.
- Overfeeding, especially carbohydrate, resulting in excess CO_2 production can exacerbate an acute respiratory acidosis. Calories should be limited to maintenance requirements.

Box 4.14 Expected Compensation, Causes, and Treatment of Respiratory Alkalosis

---

Uncompensated or Acute < 24 Hours:
- pH high (> 7.45)
- PCO_2 low (< 35 mm Hg = hypocapnia)
- HCO_3^- normal (21–28 mEq/L)

Compensated or Chronic:
- pH near normal
- PCO_2 low
- HCO_3^- low
- Renal compensation occurs through reabsorption of chloride and HCO_3^- excretion; HCO_3^- decreases approximately 4–6 mEq/L for each 10-mm Hg decrease in PCO_2.

Principal Causes:
(Hyperventilation with excess elimination of CO_2)
- Mechanical overventilation
- Central nervous system mediated: voluntary hyperventilation (anxiety, hysteria), pain; brain trauma or tumor, cerebrovascular accident
- Hypoxemia or tissue hypoxia: high altitude, severe anemia
- Pulmonary diseases: pneumonia, pulmonary embolism, pulmonary edema, interstitial lung disease, early acute respiratory distress syndrome
- Miscellaneous: pregnancy, hepatic failure, gram-negative sepsis, salicylate overdose

Treatment:
- Correct underlying disturbance
- Maintain adequate oxygenation

EFFECT OF HYDRATION ON LABORATORY VALUES

Laboratory Values and Hydration Status (2,17,21–24)

Analysis of several blood and urine indexes can offer insight into a patient's hydration status, although none will accurately predict the degree of volume deficit or excess. Interpretation requires knowledge of disease states, acid-base imbalances, and concurrent therapies that also influence laboratory results. Laboratory assessment is then used to support findings from the history and physical examination that correlate with volume depletion or excess (see Chapter 3, Nutrition-Focused Physical Assessment).

The fluid content of the body is mainly found in the intracellular (ICF) and extracellular (ECF) compartments, with a small amount of transcellular fluid within specialized cavities. The ECF is further divided into fluid within the intravascular (blood vessels), and extravascular (interstitial) spaces. *Hypovolemia*, or true volume depletion, refers to a loss of water and sodium leading to ECF volume contraction. In contrast, *dehydration* refers to the clinical consequences resulting from excessive loss of free water.

An elevated blood urea nitrogen (BUN) may suggest hypovolemia, especially if a disproportionate rise relative to creatinine is seen by a BUN/creatinine ratio that exceeds 20:1 (and other causes such as excessive protein intake or GI bleeding are ruled out). Hypovolemia resulting in decreased intravascular fluid causes hemoconcentration. The relative fluctuations in hematocrit and albumin due to intravascular plasma volume changes must be compared with the patient's baseline values. Serum sodium and osmolality are nonspecific and have the least clinical utility when viewed in isolation. Urine-specific gravity and osmolality reflect the ability of the kidneys to concentrate or dilute urine appropriately and can provide additional information when assessing hydration status.

Hypervolemia is a state of ECF volume expansion. Compared with hypovolemia, laboratory indexes are even less specific for volume changes in this condition.

Table 4.11 Laboratory Values and Hydration Status

Laboratory Test	Hypovolemia	Hypervolemia	Other Factors Influencing Lab Results
BUN Normal: 10–20 mg/dL **BUN:Creatinine ratio** Normal: 10–15:1	Increases	Decreases	**Low**—inadequate dietary protein, severe liver failure. **High**—prerenal failure, excessive protein intake, GI bleeding, catabolic state, glucocorticoid therapy. Creatinine will also rise in severe hypovolemia.
Hematocrit Normal: Male: 42%–52% Female: 37%–47%	Increases	Decreases	**Low**—anemia, hemorrhage with subsequent hemodilution (occurring after approximately 12–24 h). **High**—chronic hypoxia (chronic pulmonary disease, living at high altitude, heavy smoking), polycythemia vera, recent transfusion.

(continues next page)

Table 4.11 Laboratory Values and Hydration Status (continued)

Laboratory Test	Hypovolemia	Hypervolemia	Other Factors Influencing Lab Results
Serum albumin Normal: 3.5–5.0 g/dL	Increases	Decreases	Refer to Serum Protein section. High levels uncommon except in hemoconcentration.
Serum sodium Normal: 136–145 mEq/L	Typically increases (but can be normal or decreased)	Decreases, normal or increases	Refer to Hyponatremia and Hypernatremia in the Electrolyte section.
Serum osmolality Normal: 285–295 mOsm/kg H$_2$O	Typically increases (but can be decreased or normal)	Typically decreases (but can be increased or normal)	Refer to Hyponatremia and Hypernatremia in the Electrolyte section.
Urine-specific gravity Normal (random): 1.003–1.030	Increases	Decreases	**Low**—renal disease, diuresis, diabetes insipidus in elderly due to impaired ability to concentrate urine. **High**—glucosuria, proteinuria, excretion of radiopaque dyes.

(continues next page)

Table 4.11 Laboratory Values and Hydration Status (continued)

Laboratory Test	Hypovolemia	Hypervolemia	Other Factors Influencing Lab Results
Urine osmolality Normal: 200–1200 mOsm/kg H$_2$0	Increases	Decreases	**Low**—diuresis (osmolality decreases as urine output increases, and vice versa), diabetes insipidus, glomerulonephritis, hyponatremia, sickle cell anemia, aldosteronism. **High**—Addison's disease, azotemia, cirrhosis, glucosuria, SIADH.

NUTRITIONAL ANEMIA ASSESSMENT

Nutritional Anemias (2,3,17,28–32)

Nutritional anemias are most commonly caused by inadequate red blood cell (RBC) production due to a deficiency of iron, vitamin B-12, or folate. Laboratory values progressively change as the severity of anemia increases, with reduced hemoglobin (< 14 g/dL in men; < 12 g/dL in women) appearing in the later stages of nutrient depletion. A number of laboratory tests, along with medical and nutrition histories, are useful for detection of early deficiency and to increase the diagnostic specificity. Within 1 or 2 weeks after starting effective replacement therapy to correct a vitamin B-12—, folate-, or iron-deficiency anemia, an increased reticulocyte count would be expected because increased RBCs are produced in response to therapy.

Iron-Deficiency Anemia (IDA) and Anemia of Chronic Disease (ACD)

Although iron deficiency is the most common cause of anemia worldwide, anemia of chronic disease (ACD) may be more prevalent in the hospital setting. Several hematologic features are similar (eg, a reduced serum iron and hemoglobin (Hgb), although Hgb rarely drops below 8.0 mg/dL in ACD). Their treatments vary, however, so it is important to distinguish between these two anemias. Multiple blood tests are commonly interpreted in conjunction with a nutrition and medical history. During an acute-phase response, iron studies are altered, which must be considered when interpreting the results. If blood tests are inconclusive, a bone marrow biopsy remains the gold standard for evaluating iron stores.

Table 4.12 Diagnosis of Iron-Deficiency Anemia and Anemia of Chronic Disease

Most Useful Lab Indexes	Iron-Deficiency Anemia	Anemia of Chronic Disease[a]	Interpretation of Laboratory Tests
Serum ferritin Normal: • Men: 12–300 ng/mL • Women: 10–150 ng/mL	Decreases	Normal or increases	Serum ferritin reflects total-body iron stores. A low serum ferritin is considered diagnostic of iron deficiency and differentiates it from ACD. However, a normal ferritin level does not exclude iron deficiency, because ferritin levels are increased with an acute-phase response, liver disease, renal disease, and some cancers.
Serum iron Normal: • Men: 80–180 mcg/dL • Women: 60–160 mcg/dL	Decreases	Decreases	Serum iron represents the amount of iron in the blood where it is bound to transferrin and therefore available for RBC production. Levels are reduced in both IDA and ACD, although more markedly in severe IDA. Increases are observed in

(continues next page)

110

Table 4.12 Diagnosis of Iron-Deficiency Anemia and Anemia of Chronic Disease (continued)

Most Useful Lab Indexes	Iron-Deficiency Anemia	Anemia of Chronic Disease[a]	Interpretation of Laboratory Tests
			hemolytic states, hemachromatosis, iron overload, acute liver damage, and, transiently, after iron supplementation. Significant diurnal variation affects interpretation.
Total iron-binding capacity (TIBC) Normal: 250–460 mcg/dL	Increases	Decreases or low-normal	TIBC is an indirect measurement of serum transferrin and reflects the amount of transferrin receptors available for iron binding. A rise in TIBC above normal is typically seen in iron deficiency, as well as, blood loss, acute liver damage, and late in pregnancy. However, because transferrin is a negative acute-phase protein, it falls in any inflammatory state, even in the presence of iron deficiency (refer to Table 4.2).

(continues next page)

Table 4.12   Diagnosis of Iron-Deficiency Anemia and Anemia of Chronic Disease (continued)

Most Useful Lab Indexes	Iron-Deficiency Anemia	Anemia of Chronic Disease[a]	Interpretation of Laboratory Tests
Transferrin saturation Normal: • Men: 20%–50% • Women: 15%–50%	Decreases (< 16%–18%)	Normal or low-normal (< 20%)	Transferrin saturation indicates the extent to which transferrin is saturated with iron and, therefore, the amount of iron available to the tissues. Decreases can be seen in both IDA and ACD, but more consistently and significantly in IDA. Transferrin saturation can be calculated by (serum iron × 100%) divided by TIBC.
Red cell distribution width (RDW) Normal: 11%–14.5%	Increases	Normal	Although nonspecific, an increased RDW can be a clue for evaluation of iron deficiency. RDW begins to rise relatively early in iron deficiency, typically before a decrease in mean corpuscular volume (MCV) is observed. However, it remains normal, or near normal, in ACD.

(continues next page)

Table 4.12 Diagnosis of Iron-Deficiency Anemia and Anemia of Chronic Disease (continued)

Most Useful Lab Indexes	Iron-Deficiency Anemia	Anemia of Chronic Disease[a]	Interpretation of Laboratory Tests
Mean corpuscular volume (MCV) Normal: 80–95 fL	Decreases	Usually normal	MCV measures the average size of RBCs. It is normal in early iron deficiency, then falls as anemia progresses. However, its diagnostic value is limited, because reduced levels are also seen in approximately 15%–25% of patients with ACD.
Soluble transferrin receptor (TfR) Normal range depends on assay used	Increases	Normal	Useful to distinguish between IDA and ACD. Increased values seen in iron deficiency, hemolytic and megaloblastic anemias; myelodysplastic syndromes, and individuals living at high altitude or receiving erythropoietin therapy.

[a]ACD is an inability to use iron stores. It is typically mild and has a gradual onset, after a malignant, infectious, inflammatory or autoimmune condition. Therapy for ACD involves correcting the underlying disorder and use of erythropoietic agents. Iron supplementation is not beneficial unless a concurrent iron deficiency is present or if erythropoietin is used when the subsequent increase in RBC production requires supplemental iron. During critical illness, iron supplementation is recommended only with caution due to an increased risk of some infections.

Source: Data are from reference 32.

Vitamin B-12– and Folate-Deficiency (Megaloblastic) Anemias

The presence of hypersegmented neutrophils on the peripheral blood smear, followed by an increased MCV, is an indication of vitamin B-12 or folate deficiency. However, many patients with vitamin B-12 deficiency develop neurologic and/or psychiatric symptoms before megaloblastic anemia manifests. Serum or RBC folate and serum B-12 are commonly assessed simultaneously in an initial work-up for suspected megaloblastic anemia. It is important to determine the cause of megaloblastic anemia, because providing folic acid supplementation to a patient with B-12 deficiency will result in a transient improvement in the hematologic indexes but will allow any associated neurologic deterioration to continue.

Table 4.13 Diagnosis of Vitamin B-12– and Folate-Deficiency Anemias

Most Useful Laboratory Indexes	Vitamin B-12–Deficiency Anemia	Folate-Deficiency Anemia	Interpretation of Laboratory Tests
Mean corpuscular volume (MCV) Normal: 80–95 fL	Increases	Increases	Evaluation of the MCV alone lacks sensitivity/specificity for megaloblastic anemia, because elevations are also seen with alcoholism, liver disease, hypothyroidism, several medications, and some myelodysplastic disorders. Megaloblastic anemia is more likely if MCV is markedly elevated (> 110 fL); however, it can be normal with concurrent iron deficiency.
Serum B-12 (cobalamin) Normal: 160–950 pg/mL	Decreases	Usually normal	Interpretation of serum B-12 can be difficult, because blood levels are maintained at the expense of tissue

(continues next page)

Table 4.13 Diagnosis of Vitamin B-12– and Folate-Deficiency Anemias (continued)

Most Useful Laboratory Indexes	Vitamin B-12–Deficiency Anemia	Folate-Deficiency Anemia	Interpretation of Laboratory Tests
			stores and a specific cutoff for deficiency is controversial. For unclear reasons, up to $1/3$ of patients with folate deficiencies also have a decreased serum B-12, which rises with folate supplementation.
Serum methylmalonic acid (MMA) Normal: 73–271 nmol/L	Increases	Normal	An elevated serum MMA is very specific for vitamin B-12 deficiency; however, increases can also be seen in dehydration or renal failure. Test availability is limited.

(continues next page)

Table 4.13 Diagnosis of Vitamin B-12– and Folate-Deficiency Anemias (continued)

Most Useful Laboratory Indexes	Vitamin B-12–Deficiency Anemia	Folate-Deficiency Anemia	Interpretation of Laboratory Tests
Red blood cell (RBC) folate Normal: 150–450 ng/mL	Normal or decreases	Decreases	RBC folate reflects folate adequacy during the previous 1–3 mo. However, the test has analytic limitations and levels are reduced in patients with folate deficiency and in about 50% of patients with B-12 deficiency (because cellular uptake of folate depends on B-12).
Serum folate Normal: 5–25 ng/mL	Normal or increases	Decreases	Measurement of serum folate is common, although it may be misleading because levels fluctuate rapidly with changes in recent dietary intake. A low folate level in both plasma and RBCs is a strong indicator of deficiency.

(continues next page)

117

Table 4.13 Diagnosis of Vitamin B-12– and Folate-Deficiency Anemias (continued)

Most Useful Laboratory Indexes	Vitamin B-12–Deficiency Anemia	Folate-Deficiency Anemia	Interpretation of Laboratory Tests
Serum homocysteine Normal: 4–14 ∝mol/L	Increases greatly	Increases moderately	Increased serum homocysteine levels can be helpful but are nonspecific, because elevations are seen in folate, B-12, and B-6 deficiency or, less frequently, in renal insufficiency, hypothyroidism, and several inherited disorders or some medications.

VITAMIN, MINERAL, TRACE ELEMENT ASSESSMENT

Vitamins, Minerals, and Trace Elements (2,17,28,33–36)

Laboratory assessment can be useful to detect a subclinical nutrient deficiency or excess before physical signs manifest with some, but not all, micronutrients. An inadequate diet usually results in suboptimal status of several nutrients. However, isolated vitamin, mineral, or trace-element deficiencies can be the result of a disease state, medication interaction, or omission from PN. Inadequate iron, vitamin B-12, D, folic acid, and thiamin may be relatively common in developed countries; in developing countries, however, vitamin A, zinc, iron, and iodine are among the most commonly seen deficiencies.

The RD must be able to determine when laboratory assessment is warranted. Frequently, laboratory values can be misleading. Therefore, a thorough medical history, nutrition assessment, diet history, and knowledge of typical body nutrient stores are required to determine the likelihood of nutrient deficiency or excess. All sources of nutrients should be considered, including those found in lipid emulsions (intravenous lipid emulsions contain vitamin K as well as small amounts of phosphorus and vitamin E) and those synthesized by the body (vitamin K, biotin, and pantothenic acid from intestinal flora; vitamin D from sunlight; or niacin from tryptophan conversion).

The specific test and reference standards will vary with each laboratory's assay techniques. Interpretation can often be challenging, because results can be altered by many nonnutritional factors, notably the acute phase response (see Table 4.14).

Table 4.14 Laboratory Assessment of Selected Nutrients

Nutrient	Factors That Cause or Contribute to Deficiency	Recommended Laboratory Tests and Interpretation
Vitamin A	Fat malabsorption,ᵃ increased needs (burn, trauma, major surgery, infection), medications (oral neomycin)	*Serum retinol:* may reflect long-term vitamin A status; plasma levels are maintained until liver reserves are nearly exhausted. Decreases may also be seen in the acute-phase response, severe malnutrition, or zinc deficiency. Renal failure and oral contraceptive use may increase levels. Levels > 100 ∝g/dL (> 3.5 ∝mol/L) are commonly seen in toxicity. *Serum retinol binding protein* is a surrogate marker for retinol. Concentrations are low in vitamin A deficiency, hyperthyroidism, chronic liver disorders, an acute-phase response, and cystic fibrosis. Elevated levels occur in renal failure and acute or early liver damage.

(continues next page)

Table 4.14 Laboratory Assessment of Selected Nutrients (continued)

Nutrient	Factors That Cause or Contribute to Deficiency	Recommended Laboratory Tests and Interpretation
Vitamin D	Inadequate diet and/or inadequate skin exposure to ultraviolet light (eg, elderly or homebound individuals, especially in the winter), renal or liver failure, nephrotic syndrome, hypoparathyroidism, fat malabsorption,[a] gastrectomy, medications (anticonvulsants[b] [especially if ≥ 2], cimetidine, isoniazid, corticosteroids)	*Serum 25 hydroxyvitamin D:* requires adequate liver function for synthesis. Concentrations vary with the season, sun exposure, and vitamin D intake. Low concentrations reflect deficiency; > 200 nmol/L is potential toxicity. *Serum 1,25-dihydroxyvitamin D:* Synthesis requires adequate renal function and supply of 25 hydroxyvitamin D. Levels are typically low in deficiency; although occasionally normal as parathyroid hormone (PTH), serum calcium, and phosphate levels closely regulate production of 1.25(OH)$_2$. Levels are normal or elevated in toxicity.

(continues next page)

121

Table 4.14 Laboratory Assessment of Selected Nutrients (continued)

Nutrient	Factors That Cause or Contribute to Deficiency	Recommended Laboratory Tests and Interpretation
Vitamin D (continued)		Decreased serum phosphate and increased alkaline phosphatase and PTH are commonly seen in vitamin D deficiency; however, they are nonspecific for the diagnosis of vitamin D deficiency.
Vitamin E	Fat malabsorption,[a] abetalipoproteinemia. Increased requirements with diets very high in polyunsaturated fats.	*Plasma alpha tocopherol:* As vitamin E is transported in lipoproteins, interpretation requires an evaluation of lipid levels. If hyperlipidemia is present, use an alpha tocopherol to lipid ratio (plasma alpha-tocopherol to cholesterol mmol/L ratio < 2.2 indicates a risk of vitamin E deficiency).

(continues next page)

Table 4.14 Laboratory Assessment of Selected Nutrients (continued)

Nutrient	Factors That Cause or Contribute to Deficiency	Recommended Laboratory Tests and Interpretation
Vitamin K	Fat malabsorption,[a] liver disease (primary biliary cirrhosis), long-term PN without adequate vitamin K, medications (coumarin anticoagulants [an intentional effect], antibiotics [especially broad-spectrum and N-methylthiotetrazole– containing cephalosporins], megadoses of vitamin E, anticonvulsants, high-dose aspirin, quinine, quinidine, cyclosporine).	Prothrombin time (PT): a measure of blood clotting. It is prolonged in vitamin K deficiency but insensitive to detect subclinical deficiency unless it rapidly normalizes (beginning within hours) after intravenous supplementation. Plasma phylloquinone (K_1): reflects recent dietary intake. Increased concentrations may be seen in older age and patients with hypertriglyceridemia.
Vitamin C	Inadequate diet, increased requirements (trauma, burns, chronic infection or inflammatory diseases, smoking, pregnancy, lactation, and hyperthyroidism), dialysis, medications (barbiturates, tetracycline, high-dose aspirin).	Plasma ascorbic acid: reflects recent intake. The upper limit of 1.7 mg/dL is considered the renal threshold. Leukocyte ascorbic acid: Reflects tissue stores but is more technically difficult to perform and interpret.

(continues next page)

Table 4.14 Laboratory Assessment of Selected Nutrients (continued)

Nutrient	Factors That Cause or Contribute to Deficiency	Recommended Laboratory Tests and Interpretation
Thiamin (B-1)	Alcoholism (most common cause), refeeding syndrome, inadequate diet or omission from PN (eg, during multivitamin shortage), increased requirements (fever, pregnancy, lactation, hypermetabolism, hyperthyroidism), and dialysis medications (high-dose diuretics, prolonged antacid use).	*Erythrocyte transketolase activity (ETKA):* Can be used alone but is most sensitive/specific when thiamin pyrophosphate is added and interpreted along with a percentage of stimulation effect (TPPE). The higher the percentage stimulation (or activity coefficient), the greater the deficiency. A delay to process test results can limit its usefulness when deciding whether prompt supplementation is warranted. *Urinary thiamin:* Reflects recent intake. Requires an adequate renal conservation mechanism that decreases urinary excretion when body stores are depleted. Increased serum lactate (lactic acidosis) is a nonspecific sign of thiamin deficiency.

(continues next page)

Table 4.14 Laboratory Assessment of Selected Nutrients (continued)

Nutrient	Factors That Cause or Contribute to Deficiency	Recommended Laboratory Tests and Interpretation
Riboflavin (B-2)	Inadequate diet, alcoholism, elderly, malabsorption (celiac disease, tropical sprue), liver disease, biliary obstruction, hypothyroidism, diabetes mellitus, increased requirements (surgery, trauma, burns, pregnancy, lactation), medications (phenothiazines or tricyclic antidepressants [imipramine, amitriptyline], probenecid, chlorpromazine, adriamycin, quinocrine)	*Erythrocyte glutathione reductase activity coefficient (EGR-AC)*: a functional test reflecting riboflavin status.
Niacin (B-3)	Alcoholism, carcinoid syndrome, Hartnup's disease, malabsorption (Crohn's), medications (isoniazid, mercaptopurine). Increased requirements can be seen in cirrhosis, hypermetabolism, burns, hyperthyroidism, diabetes mellitus, pregnancy and lactation, but they rarely result in a deficient state.	Excretion of niacin metabolites in the urine is most commonly measured. *Urinary 2-pyridone* falls more precipitously than *urinary N'-methylnicotinamide.* A ratio is used if only a random urine specimen is available.

(continues next page)

125

Table 4.14   **Laboratory Assessment of Selected Nutrients** (continued)

Nutrient	Factors That Cause or Contribute to Deficiency	Recommended Laboratory Tests and Interpretation
Pyridoxine (B-6)	Alcoholism, liver disease, inadequate diet, severe riboflavin deficiency, medications (isoniazid, hydralazine, cycloserine, penicillamine, possibly oral contraceptives). Increased requirements with chronic renal failure, dialysis, pregnancy, eclampsia, preeclampsia.	*Plasma pyridoxal 5'-phosphate (PLP):* Interpretation is challenging, because it is influenced by many factors, including exercise, pregnancy, age, alkaline phosphatase levels, smoking, and some medications.
Folic acid	Inadequate diet, alcoholism, increased requirements (pregnancy, lactation, hemolytic anemia, chronic exfoliative dermatitis, dialysis), elderly, malabsorption (short bowel syndrome, celiac disease, tropical sprue), medications (sulfasalazine, folic acid antagonists,[c] pentamidine, triamterene, piritrexim, epoetin, anticonvulsants[b] [although large folic acid supplementation may reverse their effectiveness], cycloserine, possibly oral contraceptives).	*Serum folate:* indicates recent dietary intake and may not correlate with tissue stores. May be elevated in vitamin B-12 deficiency or intestinal bacterial overgrowth. *Erythrocyte (RBC) folate:* reflects intake for the life of the RBC (120 d). Simultaneous evaluation of Vitamin B-12 and homocysteine is recommended. Refer to the Anemia section.

(continues next page)

126

Table 4.14 Laboratory Assessment of Selected Nutrients (continued)

Nutrient	Factors That Cause or Contribute to Deficiency	Recommended Laboratory Tests and Interpretation
Vitamin B-12	Inadequate stomach acid (achlorhydria, autoimmune atrophic gastritis common in adults ≥ 50 years of age), inadequate intrinsic factor (pernicious anemia, gastrectomy, gastric bypass), resection or disease of the terminal ileum (short bowel syndrome, blind loop syndrome, tropical sprue), vegan diet, AIDS, medications (proton pump inhibitors,[d] H$_2$ blockers,[e] neomycin, colchicine, p-aminosalicylic acid, nitrous oxide, metformin, cholestyramine, epoetin, anticonvulsants).	*Serum cobalamin (B-12):* Most commonly used method; however, levels may be maintained at the expense of tissue stores. Elevations (including falsely high levels) can occur in myeloproliferative disorders (leukemia, lymphomas, polycythemia vera), active liver disease. *Serum methylmalonic acid (MMA):* increases early in B-12 deficiency but not in folate deficiency. Simultaneous evaluation of folic acid and homocysteine is recommended. Refer to the Anemia section.

(continues next page)

Table 4.14 Laboratory Assessment of Selected Nutrients (continued)

Nutrient	Factors That Cause or Contribute to Deficiency	Recommended Laboratory Tests and Interpretation
Pantothenic acid (B-5)	Severe prolonged malnutrition, alcoholism. Deficiency is rare and would not occur as an isolated deficiency.	*Urinary pantothenic acid (24 h):* closely related to dietary intake but varies greatly among individuals.
Biotin	PN without biotin especially in short bowel syndrome, excessive/prolonged consumption of raw egg whites, chronic hemodialysis, medications (anticonvulsants). Deficiency is rare as it is ubiquitous in the diet and produced by intestinal bacteria.	*Urinary biotin excretion:* reduced in biotin deficiency. Testing is technically demanding, and interpretation is difficult. *Urinary 3-hydroxisovalerate acid:* increased in biotin deficiency.
Iron[f]	Blood loss from GI tract (cancer, inflammatory bowel disease, ulcers, hookworm), heavy menstruation, hemodialysis; increased requirements (pregnancy, epoetin therapy),	*Serum ferritin:* falls with depletion of iron stores. Greatly elevated levels are seen in iron overload. Refer to Table 4.12. Diagnosis of Iron-Deficiency Anemia and Anemia of Chronic Disease

(continues next page)

Table 4.14 Laboratory Assessment of Selected Nutrients (continued)

Nutrient	Factors That Cause or Contribute to Deficiency	Recommended Laboratory Tests and Interpretation
Iron[f] (continued)	chronic renal failure, inadequate diet/vegetarian, long-term PN without iron, malabsorption (celiac disease, Crohn's disease, short bowel syndrome), achlorhydria (atrophic gastritis, gastrectomy, gastric bypass), medications (epoetin, chronic aspirin, proton pump inhibitors,[d] H₂ blockers[e])	*Soluble transferrin receptor (TfR):* Rises early in iron deficiency and in proportion to the magnitude of the deficit. Can help to distinguish between iron deficiency and anemia of chronic disease. Results are not affected by the acute-phase response, pregnancy, age, or gender. Test availability limited.
Zinc	Malabsorption (celiac disease, Crohn's disease, short bowel syndrome, AIDS enteropathy, large volume ileostomy, diarrhea or enteric fistula output), increased renal losses (chronic liver disease/cirrhosis, nephrotic syndrome, some cancers, diabetes, alcoholism, trauma), PN without adequate zinc, inadequate diet (high phytate/vegetarian), elderly, burns, sickle cell	*Plasma zinc:* Interpret with caution. Homeostatic mechanisms can maintain plasma concentrations for weeks despite inadequate intake. Unreliable in acute illness as decreases also correlate with degree of hypoalbuminemia and redistribution in acute-phase response. Assessment of zinc status based on hair analysis lacks clearly defined lower cut-off values.

(continues next page)

Table 4.14 Laboratory Assessment of Selected Nutrients (continued)

Nutrient	Factors That Cause or Contribute to Deficiency	Recommended Laboratory Tests and Interpretation
Zinc (continued)	anemia, acrodermatitis enteropathica, medications (penicillamine, diuretics, diethylenetriamine penta-acetate, valproate).	
Copper	PN without copper, increased losses (diarrhea, enteric fistulas, large burn wounds, nephrotic syndrome, abnormal bile loss, malabsorption (celiac disease, short bowel syndrome, tropical sprue). PCM especially recovery (although low serum levels may be due to low ceruloplasmin production), medications (penicillamine, high-dose zinc or iron). Deficiency relatively rare.	*Plasma copper or ceruloplasmin:* > 90% of copper in plasma is bound to ceruloplasmin; and changes in blood levels are usually parallel. Plasma copper is a reliable indicator of copper deficiency but does not reflect intake except when below a certain level. May not be sensitive for marginal deficiency. Refer to age- and sex-specific ranges. Increases with pregnancy, malignancy, myocardial infarction, oral contraceptive use, or an acute-phase response (as ceruloplasmin is a positive acute-phase protein). *Erythrocyte CuZn superoxide dismutase:* reflects long-term status (not commonly used).

(continues next page)

Table 4.14 Laboratory Assessment of Selected Nutrients (continued)

Nutrient	Factors That Cause or Contribute to Deficiency	Recommended Laboratory Tests and Interpretation
Selenium[f]	People in areas with low-selenium soil (China, New Zealand, Scandinavia), PN without selenium; malabsorption (prolonged diarrhea, enteric fistulas, Crohn's disease, inflammatory bowel disease, short bowel syndrome).	*Plasma selenium:* the most commonly used index of selenium status. Under steady-state conditions, it reflects intake and selenium nutriture; however, correlation with total body stores has not been established.
Chromium[f]	Long-term PN without supplementation. Requirement increased with large intestinal losses.	No reliable assay is widely available. Sample contamination is a problem. As glucose intolerance and elevated LDL cholesterol and triglycerides can be seen in chromium deficiency, improved levels after chromium supplementation have been used as an indirect indicator of chromium deficiency.
Manganese	Deficiency is extremely rare (eg, clinical tests with purified diet). Toxicity has been reported in	No sensitive and specific indicator. *Whole blood manganese:* correlates with

(continues next page)

131

Table 4.14 **Laboratory Assessment of Selected Nutrients** (continued)

Nutrient	Factors That Cause or Contribute to Deficiency	Recommended Laboratory Tests and Interpretation
Manganese (continued)	patients receiving PN, especially if biliary excretion is impaired by cholestatic disease.	magnetic resonance imaging (MRI) abnormalities and is often the most practical option. However, results are highly variable.
		Plasma manganese: assay has limited availability and is technically difficult, sample contamination is a problem, and slight hemolysis of samples can markedly increase concentration.
		Erythrocyte manganese may reflect tissue concentrations; however, it is not widely available. Toxicity may be noted by elevated blood manganese or manganese deposition in the brain, observed on MRI.
Molybdenum[f]	Rare genetic molybdenum cofactor deficiency, one reported case on long-term PN with Crohn's disease. Deficiency extremely unlikely.	Testing is difficult to perform and requires atomic absorption spectrophotometry or emission spectroscopy. Adequate assay and guidelines not available for nutrition assessment.

(continues next page)

Table 4.14 Laboratory Assessment of Selected Nutrients (continued)

Nutrient	Factors That Cause or Contribute to Deficiency	Recommended Laboratory Tests and Interpretation
Iodine[f]	Inadequate diet in endemic areas or unsupplemented food supplies; increased requirement in cold environments, stress, and with antithyroid medications. Excessive consumption of goiterogenic foods (eg, cabbage, rutabagas, broccoli, cauliflower, cassava) is usually not a clinically significant factor except with a coexisting iodine deficiency.	*Urinary iodine excretion:* used in population studies; reflects very recent intake. Ideally, obtain a 24-h urine sample. If a random sample, compare to urinary creatinine. An indirect measurement of iodine deficiency is a normal or low total thyroxine (T_4), normal or slightly elevated T_3, and a normal or only slightly elevated thyroid-stimulating hormone (TSH).

[a]Malabsorption of fat-soluble vitamins can occur with inadequate pancreatic enzymes (chronic pancreatitis, cystic fibrosis), insufficient bile salts (biliary obstruction, cholestatic liver disease), short bowel syndrome, celiac disease, Crohn's disease, tropical sprue, and medications (cholestyramine, colestipol, mineral oil, and orlistat).
[b]Common anticonvulsants include phenobarbital, phenytoin, carbamazepine, and primidone.
[c]Folate antagonists (methotrexate, pyrimethamine, trimetrexate, trimethoprim) inhibit dihydrofolate reductase inhibitors and may result in folic acid deficiency.
[d]Proton pump inhibitors include omeprazole and lansoprazole.
[e]H_2 blockers (histamine H_2-receptor antagonists) include cimetidine, ranitidine, and famotidine.
[f]Iron and iodine are not routinely added to PN. Chromium is found as a contaminant of amino acid solutions in addition to the content in the trace element package. Molybdenum and selenium are available in some trace element packages.

USING THE LABORATORY FOR MONITORING

Disease-Specific Laboratory Testing for Adults

Tables 4.15 through 4.19 describe some key uses of laboratory testing used to monitor and evaluate factors related to each nutrition diagnosis and intervention implemented by the RD. The tables are designed to illustrate laboratory testing often ordered for patients who either have or are at risk for chronic kidney disease (37,38), refeeding syndrome (3,39), essential fatty acid deficiency (40), hyperlipidemia (15,41,42), and metabolic syndrome (43). Table 4.20 explains the use of stool studies (2,17,44). These tables refer to testing for adults only.

Table 4.15 Chronic Kidney Disease

Laboratory Tests	Frequency of Monitoring and Rationale
Albumin, prealbumin	Low albumin and prealbumin are prognostic indicators of mortality risk in dialysis patients. Predialysis or stabilized[a] albumin should be measured monthly for maintenance dialysis (or every 1–3 months for nondialyzed patients with chronic renal failure), and prealbumin as needed. Goal: albumin, ≥ 4.0 mg/dL; prealbumin, ≥ 30 mg/dL. If low, assess for malnutrition.
Serum creatinine	Patients with predialysis or stabilized serum creatinine < 10 mg/dL should be assessed for malnutrition and skeletal muscle wasting.
Sodium, potassium, chloride, bicarbonate, calcium, phosphorus	Used in the assessment of fluid and acid-base imbalances, or the need for dietary alteration. Risk of soft-tissue deposition if serum calcium-phosphorus product exceeds 70 mg/dL; goal is < 55 mg^2/dL.^{2}. Bicarbonate should be measured monthly, with predialysis or stabilized levels maintained ≥ 22 mmol/L.
Hemoglobin, CBC, transferrin saturation, serum ferritin	Patients with chronic kidney disease are at high risk of anemia due to inadequate erythropoietin and iron deficiency. Assess hemoglobin at least annually. If < 13.5 g/dL (males) or < 12 g/dL (females), obtain CBC, absolute reticulocyte count, ferritin, and transferrin saturation. Monitor hemoglobin (monthly) and iron status tests (every 1–3 months) during use of erythropoiesis-stimulating agents.

(continues next page)

Table 4.15 Chronic Kidney Disease (continued)

Laboratory Tests	Frequency of Monitoring and Rationale
Fasting lipid profile	Evaluate all patients with chronic kidney disease for dyslipidemias (ie, risk of elevated TG, LDL, IDL, and VLDL, and decreased HDL). However, if total cholesterol is declining or low (< 150–180 mg/dL), screen for malnutrition is recommended.
Intact parathyroid hormone (PTH) and 25-hydroxyvitamin D	Patients with chronic kidney disease should be screened for vitamin D insufficiency/deficiency. If intact PTH is above target range, obtain baseline 25-hydroxyvitamin D measurement and, if normal, repeat annually. Algorithms for vitamin D supplementation are published elsewhere (37).
Aluminum	To evaluate the risk of aluminum toxicity, obtain serum aluminum level at least annually, and every 3 months if receiving aluminum-containing medications. Goal: < 20 mcg/L.

ᵃA predialysis measurement is obtained immediately before the initiation of a hemodialysis or intermittent peritoneal dialysis treatment. A stabilized serum measurement is obtained after the patient has stabilized on continuous ambulatory peritoneal dialysis.

Source: Data are from references 37 and 38.

Table 4.16   Risk of Refeeding Syndrome

Laboratory Tests	Frequency of Monitoring and Rationale
Potassium, phosphorus, magnesium	Initiating carbohydrate-rich nutrition after a period of starvation stimulates electrolytes to shift from the blood into the tissues for anabolism. A rapid decline in one or more of these electrolytes (K Phos, Mg), as well as sodium and water retention, is a hallmark sign of refeeding syndrome. High-risk conditions include anorexia nervosa, alcoholism, cancer cachexia, prolonged hypocaloric feeding, and profound weight loss. Baseline electrolyte concentrations are often normal, then rapidly decline upon initiation of feeding, or in some cases, electrolyte changes can be observed upon initiation of IVF containing dextrose. Take preventive actions: 1) Obtain and correct baseline electrolytes. 2) Initiate nutrition support cautiously with hypocaloric feedings (eg, 15–20 kcal/kg or $\leq$ BEE $\times$ 1.0). 3) Increase caloric intake gradually. 4) Monitor electrolytes at least daily until stable at full caloric target (typically the first 3–5 d).

Source: Data are from references 3 and 39.

Table 4.17   Essential Fatty Acid Deficiency (EFAD)

Laboratory Test	Frequency of Monitoring and Rationale
Triene (eicosatrienoic acid) to tetraene arachidonic acid) ratio	Risk factors for EFAD include severe fat malabsorption and nutrition support containing < 2%–4% of calories from linoleic acid and/or 0.25%–0.5% alpha linolenic acid. Biochemical signs of deficiency can occur within 2–4 weeks of fat-free EN or PN. Manifestation is delayed when a hypocaloric or cyclic regimen enables lipolysis of endogenous fat stores. A triene to tetraene ratio of > 0.2 confirms EFAD deficiency. Few labs process this test, which delays results.

Source: Data are from reference 40.

Table 4.18   Hyperlipidemia

Laboratory Tests	Frequency of Monitoring and Rationale
Fasting lipoprotein profile (total, LDL and HDL cholesterol, triglycerides)	• Screening for hyperlipidemia is recommended every 5 y for all persons ≥ 20 y. In patients with diabetes, lipids should be measured at least annually, except for those younger than 40 years with a low-risk profile, who should have repeat assessments every 2 years.
Classification of lipid levels in mg/dL	• LDL cholesterol: < 100 optimal, 100–129 near or above optimal, 130–159 borderline high, 160–189 high, ≥ 190 very high • Total cholesterol: < 200 desirable, 200–239 borderline high, ≥ 240 high • HDL cholesterol: < 40 low, ≥ 60 high • TG: < 150 normal; 150–199 borderline; 200–499 high; ≥ 500 very high
LDL-C goal	• High-risk patients: < 100 mg/dL (optional goal < 70 mg/dL, especially if very high risk) • Moderately high-risk patients: < 130 mg/dL • Moderate-risk patients: < 130 mg/dL • Lower risk patients: < 160 mg/dL

Source: Data are from references 15, 41, and 42.

Table 4.19   Criteria for Clinical Diagnosis of Metabolic Syndrome

Measure (any 3 of 5 constitute diagnosis of metabolic syndrome)	Categorical Cutpoints
Elevated waist circumference[a,b]	≥102 cm (≥ 40 in) in men ≥ 88 cm (≥ 35 in) in women
Elevated triglycerides	≥ 150 mg/dL or On drug treatment for elevated triglycerides[c]
Reduced HDL-C	< 40 mg/dL (1.03 mmol/L) in men < 50 mg/dL (1.3 mmol/L) in women or On drug treatment for reduced HDL-C[c]
Elevated blood pressure	≥ 130 mm Hg systolic blood pressure or ≥ 85 mm Hg diastolic blood pressure or On antihypertensive drug treatment in a patient with a history of hypertension
Elevated fasting glucose	≥ 100 mg/dL or On drug treatment for elevated glucose

[a]To measure waist circumference, locate top of right iliac crest. Place a measuring tape in a horizontal plane around abdomen at level of iliac crest. Before reading tape measure, ensure that tape is snug but does not compress the skin and is parallel to floor. Measurement is made at the end of a normal expiration.
[b]Some US adults of non-Asian origin (eg, white, black, Hispanic) with marginally increased waist circumference (eg, 94–101 cm [37–39 inches] in men and 80–87 cm [31–34 inches] in women) may have strong genetic contribution to insulin resistance and should benefit from changes in lifestyle habits, similar to men with categorical increases in waist circumference. Lower waist circumference cutpoint (eg, ≥ 90 cm [35 inches] in men and ≥ 80 cm [31 inches] in women) appears to be appropriate for Asian Americans.
[c]Fibrates and nicotinic acid are the most commonly used drugs for elevated TG and reduced HDL-C. Patients taking one of these drugs are presumed to have high TG and low HDL.

Table 4.20   Stool Studies

Laboratory Tests	*Frequency of Monitoring and Rationale*
Fecal leukocytes	The presence of fecal leukocytes (white blood cells) is a screening test for infectious or inflammatory etiologies of acute diarrhea. Positive tests are seen with bacteria that penetrate intestinal mucosa, such as *Shigella, Salmonella, Escherichia coli*, and *Campylobacter*, as well as inflammatory processes such as ulcerative colitis and antibiotic-associated colitis. Fecal leukocytes will not be present in diarrhea due to noninvasive bacteria or to viral or noninfectious causes.
Ova and parasites	Diagnosis of parasitic infection is not common in hospitalized patients unless the patient has had recent foreign travel or children in day care. Positive results are also unlikely in nosocomial diarrhea (stool specimens submitted after 3 d of hospitalization).
Clostridium difficile toxin	*Clostridium difficile*—associated diarrhea usually occurs within 1–2 mo of antibiotic use (especially clindamycin, cephalosporins, or penicillins) or occasionally chemotherapeutic agents. Diarrhea, abdominal cramps, tenderness, fever, and leukocytosis are common, although symptoms vary. Cytotoxin B is the most specific assay. If negative, 1 or 2 additional stool samples may be tested. Treatment typically includes metronidazole or oral vancomycin; antidiarrheal medications are avoided. Use of certain probiotics for prevention and treatment of antibiotic- and *clostridium difficile*—associated diarrhea may be beneficial.
Sudan stain test	This qualitative screening test for fat malabsorption can use a random stool sample. Results are reported as normal (1+), slight increase (2+), and definite increase (3+) and are only reliable for moderate to severe steatorrhea.
Fecal fat	A 72-h stool collection is obtained for a quantitative evaluation of steatorrhea. The patient should consume a diet containing 80–100 g fat/d for 1–2 days before and during the study period. Less than 7 g fat/d (or 7%) is considered normal absorption. As a coefficient of fat absorption is calculated, the test requires an accurate

(continued on next page)

Table 4.20   Stool Studies (continued)

Laboratory Tests	Frequency of Monitoring and Rationale
	record of dietary fat intake and a complete stool collection.
Fecal occult blood test	Detection of occult blood in the stool suggests blood loss (eg, GI tumors, ulcerative colitis, regional enteritis, peptic ulcer, esophageal varices, or hemorrhoids). Red meat, vegetables (turnips, horseradish), and some medications (NAIDS, iron) can cause false-positive results and Vitamin C supplementation can cause false-negative results, depending on the test used. Serial testing is used because colorectal cancers may bleed intermittently.

Source: Data are from references 2, 17, and 44.

Monitoring During Enteral and Parenteral Nutrition

Frequency of monitoring and tests ordered should be individualized based on previous laboratory data, clinical condition, and underlying disease.

Table 4.21 Acute Enteral Nutrition (EN) or Parenteral Nutrition (PN)

| | Frequency of Monitoring[a] | | |
Laboratory Tests	Baseline and Initiation	Unstable or Critically Ill Patients	Stable Hospitalized Patients
Sodium, potassium, chloride, bicarbonate	Baseline; then daily for 3 d. More frequent monitoring may be needed with refeeding syndrome.	Daily.	1–2 times/wk.
BUN, creatinine	Baseline; then daily for 3 d	Daily.	1–2 times/wk.
Glucose	Baseline; then serum or finger stick every 8 h for the first 3 d; continue until consistently < 150 mg/dL.	Daily if < 150 mg/dL. Continue every 8 h if > 150 mg/dL.	1–2 times/wk if consistently < 150 mg/dL and not requiring insulin or oral agent. Continue every 8 h if > 150 mg/dL.
Calcium	Baseline, then daily for 3 d. If low, obtain ionized calcium before considering treatment.	Daily if unstable, otherwise 2–3 times/wk.	1–2 times/wk.

(continues next page)

142

Table 4.21 Acute Enteral Nutrition (EN) or Parenteral Nutrition (PN) (continued)

Laboratory Tests	Baseline and Initiation	Unstable or Critically Ill Patients	Stable Hospitalized Patients
		Frequency of Monitoring[a]	
Phosphorus, magnesium	Baseline; then daily for 3 d. If low or risk of refeeding syndrome, monitor at least daily for 3 d or until consistently within normal range.	Daily if unstable, otherwise 2–3 times/wk.	1–2 times/wk.
Triglycerides	Baseline for PN; as medically indicated for EN.	Weekly for PN. More frequently if elevated > 400 mg/dL. As medically indicated for EN.	Weekly for PN; as medically indicated for EN.
Complete blood count (CBC) with differential[b]	Baseline for PN; as medically indicated for EN.	Weekly for PN; as medically indicated for EN.	Weekly for PN; as medically indicated for EN.

(continues next page)

Table 4.21 **Acute Enteral Nutrition (EN) or Parenteral Nutrition (PN)** (continued)

| Laboratory Tests | Baseline and Initiation | Frequency of Monitoring[a] | | |
		Unstable or Critically Ill Patients	Stable Hospitalized Patients
Aspartate aminotransferase (AST), alanine aminotransferase (ALT), alkaline phosphatase (ALP), total bilirubin	Baseline for PN; as medically indicated for EN.	1–3 times/wk for PN; as medically indicated for EN.	Weekly to monthly for PN; as medically indicated for EN.
Prothrombin time (PT), international normalized ratio (INR)	Baseline for PN; as medically indicated for EN.	Weekly for PN; as medically indicated for EN.	Weekly for PN; as medically indicated for EN.

[a]Listed for both EN and PN unless specified otherwise. Additional lab monitoring should be individualized, based on medical condition, route, tolerance to nutrition therapy, and previous lab abnormalities.

[b]Complete blood count (CBC) with differential includes: white blood cell counts (neutrophils, lymphocytes, monocytes, eosinophils, and basophils), red blood cell count, hemoglobin concentration, hematocrit, platelet count, mean corpuscular volume (MCV), mean corpuscular hemoglobin (MCH), mean corpuscular hemoglobin concentration (MCHC), and red cell distribution width (RDW).

Adapted with permission from the American Society for Parenteral and Enteral Nutrition (ASPEN) from the following: Mirtallo JM. Overview of parenteral nutrition. In: Gottschlich MM, ed. *The A.S.P.E.N. Nutrition Support Core Curriculum: A Case-Based Approach—The Adult Patient.* Silver Spring, MD: ASPEN Publishers; 2007 (reference 46); and Sacks GS, Mayhew S, Johnson D. Parental nutrition implementation and management. In: Merritt R, ed. *The A.S.P.E.N. Nutrition Support Practice Manual.* 2nd ed. Silver Spring, MD: ASPEN Publishers; 2005 (reference 47). ASPEN does not endorse the use of this material in any other form than its entirety.

Table 4.22   Home Enteral Nutrition

Laboratory Tests	Frequency of Monitoring
Sodium, potassium, chloride, glucose, BUN, creatinine, calcium, phosphorus, magnesium	Obtain baseline, then monitor until abnormalities are corrected and stable. The frequency of subsequent monitoring is based on severity of illness and is often done at routine physician visits as medically necessary based on diagnosis and during periods of EN intolerance. If stable on EN, may only need to check labs annually.
Albumin, CBC	Baseline, then as medically indicated.

Source: Data are from references 47–49.

Home Parenteral Nutrition

To evaluate tolerance and effectiveness of HPN therapy and to help minimize complications, monitor laboratory tests at regular intervals and when the clinical condition changes. Daily patient record keeping should provide information on weight, intake/output records, temperature, and urinary or blood glucose, which can alert the clinician to order additional laboratory tests to evaluate hydration status, infection, and/or glucose control. Although there are no national standards or evidence-based recommendations for routine laboratory monitoring of HPN patients, Table 4.23 provides general guidelines. Additional testing should be individualized, based on the medical condition, abnormal test results, and to assess effectiveness of changes to PN formula.

Table 4.23 — Home Parenteral Nutrition[a]

Laboratory Tests	Frequency of Monitoring
Sodium, potassium, chloride, bicarbonate glucose, BUN, creatinine, calcium, phosphorus, magnesium	Baseline, then weekly until stable, followed by monthly. Frequency may taper to quarterly (every 3 months) for stable, long-term patients.
Albumin, CBC, PT/INR	Baseline, then monthly and taper to quarterly unless medical condition warrants more frequent monitoring.
Triglyceride	Baseline, then as medically indicated if elevated or patient is at risk of hypertriglyceridemia (eg, poorly controlled diabetes, chronic renal failure, nephrotic syndrome, hypothyroidism, pancreatitis, or familial hypertriglyceridemia).
AST, ALT, ALP, GGT, total bilirubin	Baseline, then weekly for 1–2 weeks, followed by monthly for 3 months. Frequency may taper to every 3 months. ALT and AST may rise within 1–3 wks after initiation of PN and can be associated with hepatic steatosis. ALP and GGT may also rise (usually later) and may be associated with cholestasis. An elevation in total bilirubin occurs less frequently and is typically observed last.

(continues next page)

Table 4.23 Home Parenteral Nutrition[a] (continued)

Laboratory Tests	Frequency of Monitoring
Vitamins, minerals, trace elements	Optional baseline levels depending on underlying disease. Every 6 mo to annually and if clinical suspicion of deficiency or toxicity (eg, vitamins B-12, folate, 25-OH vitamin D, A, E, and C; zinc, copper, selenium, manganese, and chromium).
Iron studies (iron and ferritin)	Optional baseline levels. Every 3–6 mo if below normal or if treating for iron-deficiency anemia.
Triene:tetraene ratio	Annually in patients at risk of essential fatty acid deficiency (eg, those on lipid-free or low-lipid PN, severely malnourished, or those with physical signs/symptoms of EFAD).

[a]Patients discharged home on PN should be stable enough to require only weekly lab monitoring. Patients who have HPN started at home will initially require more frequent lab monitoring.

Source: Data are from references 50–54.

Metabolic Bone Disease

Patients receiving long-term HPN should be monitored for metabolic bone disease. Evaluate bone mineral density using dual-energy x–ray absorptiometry (DXA) every 1 to 2 years. Monitor serum calcium, phosphorus, and magnesium to maintain normal serum concentrations. Obtain a 24-hour urine collection for calcium and magnesium every 6 to 12 months. Monitor baseline serum 25 OH vitamin D and intact PTH annually or as needed (51,53).

REFERENCES

1. American Dietetic Association. *Nutrition Diagnosis: A Critical Step in the Nutrition Care Process*. Chicago, IL: American Dietetic Association; 2006.

2. Pagana KD, Pagana TJ. *Mosby's Manual of Diagnostic and Laboratory Tests*. 3rd ed. St Louis, Mo: Mosby; 2006.

3. Russell MK. Laboratory monitoring. In: Matarese LE, Gottschlich MM, eds. *Contemporary Nutrition Support Practice: A Clinical Guide*. 2nd ed. St. Louis, MO: WB Saunders; 2003:45–62.

4. Fuhrman MP, Charney P, Mueller CM. Hepatic proteins and nutrition assessment. *J Am Diet Assoc*; 2004;104:1258–1264.

5. Charney P. Nutrition assessment in the intensive care unit: prealbumin, c-reactive protein, or none of the above? *Support Line*. 2007;29:13–18.

6. Vincent JL, Dubois MJ, Navickis RJ, Wilkes MM. Hypoalbuminemia in acute illness: is there a rationale for intervention? A meta-analysis of cohort studies and controlled trials. *Ann Surg*. 2003;237:319–334.

7. Russell MK, Mueller C. Nutrition screening and assessment. In: Gottschlich MM, ed. *The A.S.P.E.N. Nutrition Support Core Curriculum: A Case-Based Approach—The Adult Patient*. Silver Spring, MD: ASPEN; 2007:163–186.

8. The Expert Committee on the Diagnosis and Classification of Diabetes Mellitus. American Diabetes Association: clinical practice recommendations 2007. *Diabetes Care*. 2007;30(Suppl 1):S1–S103. Also available at: http://care.diabetesjournals.org/content/vol30/suppl_1.

9. American Diabetes Association. Diagnosis and classification of diabetes mellitus. *Diabetes Care*. 2007;30(Suppl 1):S42-S47.

10. Nasraway SA. Hyperglycemia during critical illness. *JPEN J Parenter Enteral Nutr*. 2006;30:254–258.

11. Van den Berghe G, Wouters P, Weekers F, Verwaest C, Bruyninckx F, Schetz M, Vlasselaers D, Ferdinande P, Lauwers P, Bouillon R. Intensive insulin therapy in the critically ill patients. *N Engl J Med*. 2001;345:1359–1367.

12. Van den Berghe G, Wilmer A, Hermans G, Meersseman W, Wouters PJ, Milants I, Van Wijngaerden E, Bobbaers H, Bouillon R. Intensive insulin therapy in the medical ICU. *N Engl J Med*. 2006;354:449–461.

13. American Diabetes Association. Standards of medical care in diabetes–2006. *Diabetes Care*. 2006;29(Suppl):S4–42.

14. AACE Diabetes Mellitus Clinical Practice Guidelines Task Force. American Association of Clinical Endocrinologists medical guidelines for clinical practice for the management of diabetes mellitus. *Endocr Pract*. 2007;13(Suppl 1):3–68.

15. Buse JB, Ginsberg HN, Bakris GL, Clark NG, Costa F, Eckel R, Fonseca V, Gerstein HC, Grundy S, Nesto RW, Pignone MP, Plutzky J, Porte D, Redberg R, Stitzel KF, Stone NJ; American Heart Association; American Diabetes Association. Primary prevention of cardiovascular diseases in people with diabetes mellitus: a scientific statement from the American Heart Association and the American Diabetes Association. *Diabetes Care*. 2007; 30:162–172.

16. Nathan DM, Cleary PA, Backlund JY, Genuth SM, Lachin JM, Orchard TJ, Raskin P, Zinman B; Diabetes Control and Complications Trial/Epidemiology of Diabetes Interventions and Complications (DCCT/EDIC) Study Research Group. Intensive diabetes treatment and cardiovascular disease in patients with type 1 diabetes. *N Engl J Med*. 2005;353:2643–2653.

17. Kee JL, ed. *Laboratory and Diagnostic Tests with Nursing Implications*. 7th ed. Upper Saddle River, NJ: Pearson Prentice Hall. 2005.

18. American Diabetes Association. Standards of care in diabetes–2007. *Diabetes Care*. 2007;30(suppl 1):S4-S41.

19. American Diabetes Association. Position statement. Hyperglycemic crises in diabetes. *Diabetes Care*. 2004;27(Suppl 1):S92-S102. Also available at: http://care.diabetesjournals.org/content/vol27/suppl_1/index.shtml. Accessed November 11, 2007.

20. American Diabetes Association. Hyperglycemic crises in diabetes. *Diabetes Care*. 2004;27(Suppl 1):S94-S102.

21. Heusel JW, Siggaard-Andersen O, Scott MG. Physiology and disorders of water, electrolyte, and acid-base metabolism. In: Burtis CA, Ashwood ER, eds. *Tietz Fundamentals of Clinical Chemistry*. 5th ed. Philadelphia, PA: WB Saunders; 2001:723–745.

22. Narins RG, Jones ER, Stom MC, Rudnick MR, Bastl CP. Diagnostic strategies in disorders of fluid, electrolyte and acid-base homeostasis. *Am J Med*. 1982;72:496–520.

23. Singer GG, Brenner BM. Fluid and electrolyte disturbances. In: Kasper DL, Fauci AS, Longo DL, Braunwald E, Hauser SL, Jameson JL, eds. *Harrison's Principles of Internal Medicine*. 17th ed. New York, NY: McGraw-Hill; 2005:252–263.

24. Whitmire SJ. Fluids, electrolytes and acid-base balance. In: Matarese LE, Gottschlich MM, eds. *Contemporary Nutrition Support Practice: A Clinical Guide*. 2nd ed. Philadelphia, PA: WB Saunders; 2003:127–144.

25. Avner ED. Clinical disorders of water metabolism: hyponatremia and hypernatremia. *Pediatr Ann*. 1995;24:23–30.

26. Dickerson RN, Alexander KH, Minard G, Croce MA, Brown RO. Accuracy of methods to estimate ionized and "corrected" serum calcium concentrations in critically ill multiple trauma patients receiving specialized nutrition support. *JPEN J Parenter Enteral Nutr*. 2004;28:133–41.

27. Simmons JF, Assell CC. Acid-base basics. *Support Line*. 2001;23:6–11.

28. Boosalis MG. Micronutrients. In: Gottschlich MM, Fuhrman MP, Hammond KA, Holcombe BJ, Seidner DL, eds. *The Science and Practice of Nutrition Support: A Case-Based Core Curriculum*. Dubuque, IA: Kendall/Hunt; 2001:85–106.

29. Brittenham GM. Disorders of iron metabolism: iron deficiency and overload. In: Hoffman R, Benz EJ, Shattil SJ, Furie B, Cohen HJ, Silberstein LE, McGlave P, eds. *Hematology: Basic Principles and Practice*. 3rd ed. New York, NY; 2000:397–418.

30. Klee GG. Cobalamin and folate evaluation: measurement of methylmalonic acid and homocysteine vs vitamin B-12 and folate. *Clin Chem*. 2000;46:1277–1283.

31. Killip S, Bennet JM, Chambers MD. Iron Deficiency Anemia. *Am Fam Physician*. 2007;75:671–678.

32. DeBellis RJ. Anemia in critical care patients: incidence, etiology, impact, management, and use of treatment guidelines and protocols. *Am J Health Syst Pharm.* 2007;64(3 Suppl 2):S14-S21.

33. McCormick DB, Klee GG. Vitamins. In: Burtis CA, Ashwood ER, eds. *Tietz Fundamentals of Clinical Chemistry.* 5th ed. Philadelphia, PA: WB Saunders; 2001:543–567.

34. Heimburger DC, McLaren DS, Shils ME. Clinical manifestations of human vitamin and mineral deficiencies and toxicities: a resume. In: Shils ME, Shike M, Ross AC, Caballero B, Cousins RJ, eds. *Modern Nutrition in Health and Disease.* 10th ed. Philadelphia, PA: Lippincott Williams & Wilkins; 2006:595–612.

35. Sauberlich HE: *Laboratory Tests for the Assessment of Nutritional Status.* 2nd ed. New York, NY: CRC Press; 1999.

36. Institute of Medicine. *Dietary Reference Intakes for Vitamin A, Vitamin K, Arsenic, Boron, Chromium, Copper, Iodine, Iron, Manganese, Molybdenum, Nickel, Silicon, Vanadium, and Zinc.* Washington, DC: National Academy Press; 2001. http://www.nap.edu/openbook.php?record_id=10026&page=442. Accessed October 26, 2007.

37. Bailie GR, Johnson CA, Mason NA, St. Peter WL, eds. Chronic Kidney Disease 2006: A Guide to Select NKF-KDOQI Guidelines and Recommendations. http://www.kidney.org/professionals/kls/pdf/Pharmacist_CPG.pdf. Accessed October 23, 2007.

38. National Kidney Foundation. K/DOQI clinical practice guidelines and clinical practice recommendations for anemia in chronic kidney disease. *Am J Kidney Dis.* 2006;47 (Suppl 3): S1–S146. http://www.kidney.org/professionals/kdoqi/guidelines_anemia/index.htm. Accessed October 18, 2007.

39. McCray S, Walker S, Parrish CR. Much ado about refeeding. *Pract Gastroenterol.* 2005(Jan):26–41. http://www.healthsystem.virginia.edu/internet/digestive-health/nutrition/resources.cfm. Accessed November 20, 2007.

40. Hise ME, Brown JC. Lipids. In: Gottschlich MM, ed. *The A.S.P.E.N. Nutrition Support Core Curriculum: A Case-Based Approach—the Adult Patient.* Silver Spring, MD: A.S.P.E.N.; 2007:48–70.

41. Expert Panel on Detection, Evaluation, and Treatment of High Blood Cholesterol in Adults. Executive summary of the third report of the National Cholesterol Education Program (NCEP)

expert panel on detection, evaluation, and treatment of high blood cholesterol in adults (adult treatment panel III). *JAMA.* 2001;285:2486–2509.

42. Grundy SM, Cleeman JI, Merz CNB, Brewer HB, Clark LT, Hunninghake DB, Pasternak RC, Smith SC Jr, Stone NJ; National Heart, Lung, and Blood Institute; American College of Cardiology Foundation; American Heart Association. Implications of recent clinical trials for the national cholesterol education program adult treatment panel III guidelines. *Circulation.* 2004;110:227–239.

43. Grundy SM, Cleeman JI, Daniels SR, Donato KA, Eckel RH, Franklin BA, Gordon DJ, Krauss RM, Savage PJ, Smith SC Jr, Spertus JA, Costa F; American Heart Association; National Heart, Lung, and Blood Institute. Diagnosis and management of the metabolic syndrome. An American Heart Association/ National Heart, Lung, and Blood Institute scientific statement (errata in *Circulation.* 2005;112;e298). *Circulation.* 2005; 112:2735–2752.

44. McFarland LV. Meta-analysis of probiotics for the prevention of antibiotic associated diarrhea and the treatment of *clostridium difficile* disease. *Am J Gastroenterol.* 2006;101:812–822.

45. Mirtallo JM. Overview of parenteral nutrition. In: Gottschlich MM, ed. *The A.S.P.E.N. Nutrition Support Core Curriculum: A Case-Based Approach—The Adult Patient.* Silver Spring, MD: ASPEN Publishers; 2007.

46. Sacks GS, Mayhew S, Johnson D. Parental nutrition implementation and management. In: Merritt R, ed. *The A.S.P.E.N. Nutrition Support Practice Manual.* 2nd ed. Silver Spring, MD: ASPEN Publishers; 2005.

47. Ireton-Jones CS. Home enteral nutrition support in adults. In: Ireton-Jones CS, DeLegge MH, eds. *Handbook of Home Nutrition Support.* Sudbury, MA: Jones and Bartlett Publishers; 2007:83–101.

48. Pattinson A, Buchholtz J. Home enteral nutrition. In: Charney P, Malone A, eds. *ADA Pocket Guide to Enteral Nutrition.* Chicago, IL: American Dietetic Association; 2006:193–227.

49. Kovacevich DS, Orr ME. Considerations for home nutrition support. In: Merritt R, ed. *The A.S.P.E.N. Nutrition Support Practice Manual.* 2nd ed. Silver Spring, MD: ASPEN Publishers; 2005:371–377.

50. DeLegge MH, Ireton-Jones C. Home care. In: Gottschlich MM, ed. *The A.S.P.E.N. Nutrition Support Core Curriculum: A Case-Based Approach—the Adult Patient.* Silver Spring, MD: ASPEN Publishers; 2007:725–739.

51. Hamilton C, Seidner DL. Home parenteral nutrition in adults. In: Ireton-Jones CS, DeLegge MH, eds. *Handbook of Home Nutrition Support.* Sudbury, MA: Jones and Bartlett Publishers; 2007:115–152.

52. Hamilton C, Austin T. Home parenteral nutrition. In: Charney P, Malone A, eds. *ADA Pocket Guide to Parenteral Nutrition.* Chicago, IL: American Dietetic Association; 2007:118–146.

53. Kelly DG. Guidelines and available products for parenteral vitamins and trace elements. *JPEN J Parenter Enteral Nutr.* 2002:26(5 Suppl):S34-S36.

54. Furhman MP. Micronutrient assessment in long-term home parenteral nutrition patients. *Nutr Clin Pract.* 2006;21:566–575.

chapter 5

Anthropometric Assessment

JENNIFER LEFTON, MS, RD, CNSD, AND
AINSLEY M. MALONE, MS, RD, CNSD

Anthropometric measurements include various measures
of body weight, size, and composition used to evaluate
nutritional status. They are useful in monitoring the need
for, and effects of, nutrition intervention for disease,
trauma, and malnutrition.

HAMWI METHOD FOR IDEAL BODY WEIGHT

Equations

To calculate ideal body weight (IBW), also known as
desirable body weight (DBW), the following formulas
may be used (1).

1. IBW in Pounds and Inches
Men: 106 pounds for the first 5 feet
          Plus 6 pounds for every inch thereafter
Women: 100 pounds for the first 5 feet
          Plus 5 pounds for every inch thereafter

2. IBW in Kilograms and Meters
Men: 48.1 kg for each 1.52 m
          Plus 0.9 kg for every centimeter above 1.52 m
Women: 45.5 kg for each 1.52 m
          Plus 1.1 kg for every centimeter above 1.52 m

Example

IBW for a man who is 6 feet, 3 inches tall (15 inches above 5 feet)

$$IBW = 106 + (6 \times 15) \text{ pounds}$$
$$= 106 + 90 \text{ pounds}$$
$$= 196 \text{ pounds}$$

Adjustments for Body Frame Size

For both the metric and nonmetric formulas, 10% can be added or subtracted to the final value to accommodate variations in body frame size.

Use in Obesity

Adjusting the ideal body weight for the obese patient is controversial. Although some clinicians use such an adjustment, scientific validation for this practice is lacking. It is therefore not included here.

Adjustment for Spinal Cord Injury (2)

Paraplegia: Subtract 5% to 10% from IBW
Quadriplegia: Subtract 10% to 15% from IBW

ESTIMATING STATURE

Nonambulatory persons and those with contractures, paralysis, or other conditions limiting their ability to stand will require an estimation of their height.

Knee Height

Refer to reference 3 for measurement procedure.

- Measurement is taken with the subject in a supine position using the left leg.
- A sliding caliper is required.

- The knee and ankle should be positioned at a 90° angle.

Men:

Stature (cm) = $[2.02 \times \text{knee height (cm)}] - (0.04 \times \text{age}) + 64.19$

Women:

Stature (cm) = $[1.83 \times \text{knee height (cm)}] - (0.24 \times \text{age}) + 84.88$

Arm Span (4)

Measurement is taken from the sternal notch to the longest finger on the dominant hand. To estimate stature, multiply the number obtained by 2.

Reliable measurements may be difficult in those individuals with contractures or spinal deformities and in those who are unable to fully extend their arms.

BODY MASS INDEX (QUETELET'S INDEX) (5)

Body mass index (BMI) is a ratio of weight to height and is used as an estimate of body fat in the healthy population. (See BMI classification in Table 5.1 [6,7].)

Table 5.1   Body Mass Index Classification

BMI	Classification
≥ 40	Obesity—grade III
35–39.9	Obesity—grade II
30–34.9	Obesity—grade I
25-29.9	Overweight
18.5–24.9	Normal
< 18.4	Underweight

Source: Data are from references 6 and 7.

Equations

BMI can be calculated using the following equations:

1. $\text{BMI} = \dfrac{\text{Weight (kg)}}{\text{Height (m}^2)}$

2. $\text{BMI (kg/m}^2) = \text{pounds} \div \text{inches} \div \text{inches} \div 0.0014192$

3. $703.1 \times \dfrac{\text{Weight (lb)}}{\text{Height (in)}^2}$

Examples

1. Use formula 1 for an individual 6 feet, 3 inches (1.9 m) in height, 208 pounds (94.5 kg):

    $\text{BMI} = 94.5 \div (1.9 \times 1.9) = 94.5 \div 3.61 = 26.2$

    Classified as Overweight (see Table 5.1)

2. Use formula 2 for an individual 6 feet, 3 inches in height, 208 pounds:

    $\text{BMI} = 208 \div 75 \div 75 \div 0.0014192 = 26$

    Classified as Overweight

3. Use formula 3 for an individual 6 feet, 3 inches (75 inches), 208 pounds:

    $\text{BMI} = (703.1 \times 208) \div (75 \times 75)$
    $= 146.244.8 \div 5625 = 26$

    Classified as Overweight

Interpretation and Applicability in Special Populations

The use of BMI has not been validated in acutely ill patients. However, BMI is frequently used in the assessment of acutely ill patients and may be one of several potential indicators leading to a nutrition diagnosis (8). Results must be interpreted individually.

The correlation between BMI and body fatness is less accurate in those with an increased percentage of fat-free mass (eg, athletes) or with fluid imbalances (eg, edema). Additionally, mortality is not increased in older adults with a BMI result that is considered overweight and some contend that the normal weight BMI range may be too restrictive when used for the elderly (9).

WAIST CIRCUMFERENCE

Waist circumference assesses abdominal fat content and is measured around the smallest area below the rib cage and above the umbilicus (10). BMI and waist circumference highly correlate with obesity and risk for disease, and both measures should be used to classify overweight/obesity and to estimate disease risk (11). A waist circumference greater than 40 cm for men and greater than 35 cm for women is considered a risk factor for disease.

PERCENTAGE OF IDEAL/DESIRABLE BODY WEIGHT AND USUAL BODY WEIGHT (12)

Equations

The following formula can be used to calculate percentage of ideal body weight (IBW), also known as desirable body weight (DBW):

$$\% \text{ IBW or DBW} = \frac{\text{Current Body Weight (CBW)}}{\text{IBW or DBW}} \times 100\%$$

To calculate percentage of "usual" body weight (UBW), use the following equation:

$$\% \text{ UBW} = \frac{\text{Current Weight}}{\text{UBW}} \times 100\%$$

Examples

1. Calculate % IBW for an individual with IBW of 166 lb and CBW of 142 lb:

    $\frac{142 \text{ lb}}{166 \text{ lb}} \times 100\% = 86\% \text{ of IBW}$

2. Calculate % UBW for a patient whose weight decreased from 129 lb to 101 lb in 6 months (UBW = 129 lb; CBW = 101 lb):

    $\frac{101 \text{ lb}}{129 \text{ lb}} \times 100\% = 78\% \text{ of UBW}$

Interpretation

Refer to Table 5.2 for guidelines for interpreting % IBW and % UBW.

Table 5.2   Assessment of Body Weight

Index	Mild Deficit, %	Moderate Deficit, %	Severe Deficit, %
Ideal body weight	80–90	70–79	< 70
Usual body weight	85–95	75–84	< 75

PERCENTAGE OF WEIGHT CHANGE (12)

Equation

$$\% \text{ Weight Change} = \frac{\text{UBW} - \text{CBW}}{\text{UBW}} \times 100$$

Example

A patient's weight decreased from 129 lb to 101 lb in 6 months.

$$\frac{129 \text{ lb} - 101 \text{ lb}}{129 \text{ lb}} \times 100$$

$$\frac{28 \text{ lb}}{129 \text{ lb}} = .22 \times 100 = 22\% \text{ weight change}$$

Interpretation

Refer to Table 5.3 for guidelines for interpreting % weight change.

Table 5.3   Assessment of Weight Change

Time Period of Weight Change	Significant % Weight Loss	Severe % Weight Loss
1 wk	1–2	> 2
1 mo	5	> 5
3 mo	7.5	> 7.5
6 mo	10	>10

WEIGHT OF SELECTED BODY COMPONENTS (13)

When estimating IBW, it is necessary to account for the missing body component(s). Use the following formula and the percentages shown in Table 5.4 to estimate IBW accounting for missing body component:

Estimated IBW =
$$\frac{100 - \% \text{ amputation}}{100} \times \text{IBW for original height}$$

**Table 5.4 Percentage of Body Weight
Contributed by Specific Body Parts**

Body Part	Percentage
Trunk w/o limbs	50.0
Hand	0.7
Forearm with hand	2.3
Forearm w/o hand	1.6
Upper arm	2.7
Entire arm	5.0
Foot	1.5
Lower leg with foot	5.9
Lower leg w/o foot	4.4
Thigh	10.1
Entire leg	16.0

Example

Estimate IBW in a patient status post a below-the-knee amputation (original IBW = 166 lb). Lower leg with foot = 5.9% of total-body weight.

$$\text{Estimated IBW} = \frac{100\% - 5.9\%}{100\%} \times 166 \text{ lb}$$

$$= \frac{94.1\%}{100\%} \times 166 = .941 \times 166 = 156 \text{ lb}$$

MEASUREMENT OF BODY COMPOSITION (14)

Estimations of fat-free and fat mass in the hospitalized patient may be useful in identifying the presence of malnutrition. Triceps skinfold measurement is an index of body fat stores; arm muscle area represents muscle protein.

The limitations in using these measurements in the hospitalized patient include the following:

- Inexperienced clinicians performing measurements
- Alterations in a patient's hydration status
- Variation in body composition of selected populations (eg, athletes)
- Lack of appropriate standards for the hospitalized population

Anthropometric and Derived Anthropometric Parameters

The following are anthropometric parameters for body composition:

- Triceps skinfold thickness (TSF)
- Mid- to upper-arm circumference (AC)

The following are derived anthropometric parameters of body composition:

- Mid-upper arm fat area (AFA)
- Arm muscle area (AMA)

Equations to Calculate Derived Parameters (15)

AFA and AMA are based on measurements of TSF and AC. The following four equations to correct for bone area are used to allow a more accurate assessment of bone-free muscle area.

1. To determine total upper arm area (TAA):

$$\text{TAA (cm}^2) = \frac{AC^2}{4 \times 3.14}$$

2. To determine uncorrected AMA:

$$\text{AMA (cm}^2) = \frac{[AC - (TSF \times 3.14)]^2}{4 \times 3.14}$$

3. To determine corrected AMA (AMAc):

$$AMAc\ Males = AMA - 10\ cm^2$$

$$AMAc\ Females = AMA - 6.5\ cm^2$$

4. To determine AFA as the difference between TAA and uncorrected AMA:

$$AFA\ (cm^2) = TAA - AMA$$

Examples

1. Calculation of TAA for individual with AC of 30 cm:

$$TAA = \frac{30^2}{12.57} = 71.6\ cm^2$$

2. Calculation of uncorrected AMA for individual with AC of 30 cm and TSF of 25 mm:

$$AMA = \frac{[30 - (2.5 \times 3.14)]^2}{4 \times 3.14}$$

$$= \frac{490.44}{12.57}$$

$$= 39\ cm^2$$

3a. Calculation of corrected AMA for man with AMA of 39 cm²:

$$AMAc = 39\ cm^2 - 10\ cm^2 = 29\ cm^2$$

3b. Calculation of corrected AMA for woman with AMA of 39 cm²:

$$AMAc = 39\ cm^2 - 6.5\ cm^2 = 32.5\ cm^2$$

4. Calculation of AFA for individual with TAA of 71.6 and AMA of 39.0:

$$AFA = 71.6 - 39.0 = 32.6\ cm^2$$

Interpretation of AFA and AMA

After they are calculated, AFA and AMA are then compared with reference data (16) to determine a percentile rank. See Table 5.5 for the interpretation of arm muscle and fat areas reflecting alterations in total-body weight. The reference data (16) represent measurements obtained from samples from noninstitutionalized adults in the First and Second National Health and Nutrition Examination Surveys (NHANES 1 and NHANES 2). Ethnic variability within the samples is lacking. Using skinfold measurements in these populations may not be valid. Performing serial measurements of body composition may be useful for assessing long-term changes in fat mass and fat-free mass in chronically ill patients and/or those being repleted with enteral or parenteral nutrition.

Table 5.5   Arm Muscle and Fat Areas Reflecting Alterations in Total-Body Weight

Percentile Rank	AMA	AFA	Total-Body Weight
< 5	Muscle deficit	Fat deficit	Total-body wasting
5.1–15	Below average	Below average	Below average
15.1–85	Average	Average	Average
> 85	Above-average musculature	Excess fat	Excess total-body weight

Abbreviations: AMA, arm muscle area; AFA, Mid-upper arm fat area.

REFERENCES

1. Hamwi GJ. Changing dietary concepts. In: Donowski TS, ed. *Diabetes Mellitus: Diagnosis and Treatment.* New York, NY: American Diabetes Association; 1964:73–78.

2. Peiffer SC, Blust P, Leyson JF. Nutritional assessment of the spinal cord injured patient. *J Am Diet Assoc.* 1981;78:501–505.

3. Chumlea WC, Roche AF, Steinbaugh ML. Estimating stature from knee height for persons 60–90 years of age. *J Am Geriatr Soc.* 1985;33:116–120.

4. Mitchell CO, Lipschitz DA. Arm length measurement as an alternative to height in the nutritional assessment of the elderly. *JPEN J Parenter Enteral Nutr.* 1982;6:226–229.

5. Lee RD, Nieman DC. Anthropometry. In: *Nutritional Assessment.* Boston, MA: McGraw Hill; 1996:223–288.

6. Heymsfield SB, Baumgartner RN, Pan SF. Nutritional assessment of malnutrition by anthropometric methods. In: Shils ME, Olson JA, Shike M, Ross AC, eds. *Modern Nutrition in Health and Disease.* Baltimore, MD: Williams and Wilkins; 1999:903–921.

7. Obesity Education Initiative Task Force. *Clinical Guidelines on the Identification, Evaluation, and Treatment of Overweight and Obesity in Adults.* Washington, DC: National Institutes of Health; 1998.

8. *Nutrition Diagnosis and Intervention: Standardized Language for the Nutrition Care Process.* Chicago, IL: American Dietetic Association; 2007.

9. Heiat A, Vaccarino V, Krumholz HM. An evidence-based assessment of federal guidelines for overweight and obesity as they apply to elderly patients. *Arch Intern Med.* 2001;161:1194–1203.

10. Hammond KA. Assessment: dietary and clinical data. In: Mahan LK, Escott-Stump S, eds. *Krause's Food, Nutrition, & Diet Therapy.* 12th ed. Philadelphia, PA: Saunders; 2004:383–410.

11. American Dietetic Association Evidence Analysis Library. Adult Weight Management Guidelines. http://www.adaevidence library.com. Accessed April 5, 2007.

12. Blackburn GL, Bistrian BR. Nutritional and metabolic assessment of the hospitalized patient. *JPEN J Parenter Enteral Nutr.* 1977;1:11–22.

13. Osterkamp LK. Current perspective on assessment of human body proportions of relevance to amputees. *J Am Diet Assoc.* 1995;95:215–218.

14. Lee RD, Nieman DC. Assessment of the hospitalized patient. In: *Nutritional Assessment.* Boston, MA: McGraw Hill; 1996:289–331.

15. Howell WH. Anthropometry and body composition analysis. In: Gottschlich MM, Matarese LE, eds. *Contemporary Nutrition Support Practice: A Clinical Guide.* 2nd ed. Philadelphia, PA: WB Saunders; 2003:31–44.

16. Frisancho AR. *Anthropometric Standards for the Assessment of Growth and Nutritional Status.* Ann Arbor, MI: University of Michigan Press; 1990.

chapter 6

Nutrient Requirements

Mary Russell, MS, RD, CNSD, and
Ainsley M. Malone, MS, RD, CNSD

ENERGY REQUIREMENTS

Several methods exist for estimating energy requirements. Deciding which method to use is frequently based on the patient's clinical status and available patient data. In 2007, the American Dietetic Association (ADA) completed evidence analyses of various methods for determining energy requirements to help clarify which methods are most closely aligned to actual energy expenditure (1). The information provided separates estimation of energy requirements into three sections: the acutely ill patient, the critically ill patient, and the patient who is obese (with a body mass index [BMI] ≥ 30).

ENERGY REQUIREMENTS
FOR ACUTELY ILL PATIENTS

Mifflin-St. Jeor Equation

According to ADA's Evidence Analysis Library (2), "estimated energy needs should be based on RMR [resting metabolic rate]. If possible, RMR should be measured (eg, indirect calorimetry). If RMR cannot be measured, the Mifflin-St. Jeor equation using actual weight is the most accurate for estimating RMR for overweight and obese individuals. *Strong, Conditional*."

The Mifflin-St. Jeor equations are as follows (3):

Men: RMR = 5 + 10W + 6.25 H − 5A

Women: RMR = 161 + 10W + 6.25H − 5A

Where: RMR = resting metabolic rate (energy expenditure) in kilocalories; W = weight in kilograms; H = height in centimeters; A = age in years.

Ireton-Jones Equation (1997)

The following Ireton-Jones equation (4) calculates estimated energy expenditure for spontaneously breathing patients. This equation is part of two equations that were derived from hospitalized patients with different clinical states (diabetes, pancreatitis, trauma, and burns) and have been validated.

EEE = 629 − 11(A) + 25(W) − 609(O)

Where: EEE = estimated energy expenditure (kcal/d); A = age (years); W = weight (kg); O = presence of obesity > 30% above ideal body weight (0 = absent; 1 = present); G = gender (female = 0; male = 1); T = diagnosis of trauma (absent = 0; present = 1); B = diagnosis of burn (absent = 0; present = 1).

ENERGY REQUIREMENTS FOR CRITICALLY ILL PATIENTS

Indirect Calorimetry

Indirect calorimetry uses measurements of inspired and expired gas volumes to indirectly calculate energy expenditure. Requirements for a valid measurement include the following:

- Hemodynamically stable patient
- Cooperative or sedated patient
- Period of rest before measurement
- $FiO_2 < 60\%$
- Absence of chest tubes or other sources of air leak
- Absence of supplemental oxygen
- Absence of hyperventilation

This method is frequently recommended as the "gold standard" for assessing energy requirement as it most closely relates to actual energy expenditure and it accounts for variability in energy expenditure from changes in metabolic state. However, limitations in its use can be significant. These include its expense as a method of indirectly measuring energy expenditure, the need for technical expertise to operate equipment and interpret test results and concerns regarding validity in specific patients (see requirements).

According to the ADA Evidence Analysis Library (5), "Indirect calorimetry is the standard for determination of RMR in critically ill patients since RMR based on measurement is more accurate than estimation using predictive equations. *Strong, Imperative.*"

Respiratory Quotient

Respiratory quotient, a measure of carbon dioxide produced over oxygen consumed, has historically been used to evaluate substrate utilization.

According to the ADA Evidence Analysis Library (6), "if RQ is below 0.7 or above 1.0, then repeated measures are necessary under more optimal conditions. An RQ under 0.70 suggests hypoventilation (inadequate removal of metabolic carbon dioxide from the blood to the lung) or prolonged fasting. An RQ above 1.0, in the absence of overfeeding, suggests hyperventilation (removal of carbon dioxide from the blood to the lung in excess of the amount produced by metabolism) or inaccurate gas collection. *Strong, Conditional.*"

Predictive Equations

Predictive equations have been developed as an alternative to indirect calorimetry for assessing energy requirements.

According to ADA's Evidence Analysis Library (5), "if predictive equations are needed in nonobese, critically ill patients, consider using one of the following, as they have the best prediction accuracy of equations studied (listed in order of accuracy): Penn State, 2003a (79%), Swinamer (55%) and Ireton-Jones, 1992 (52%). In some individuals, errors between predicted and actual energy needs will result in under- or over-feeding. *Fair, Conditional.*"

The ADA Evidence Analysis Library (5) also concludes that "the Harris-Benedict (with or without activity and stress factors), the Ireton-Jones, 1997, and the Fick [equations] should not be considered for use in RMR determination in critically ill patients, as these equations do not have adequate prediction accuracy. In addition, the Mifflin-St. Jeor equation should not be considered for use in critically ill patients, as it was developed for healthy people and has not been well researched in the critically ill population. *Strong, Imperative.*"

Penn State Equation for Resting Metabolic Rate (2003a)

The Penn State equation (2003a) is as follows (7):

$$RMR = BMR(0.85) \times V_E(33) + T_{max}(175) - 6433$$

Where: BMR = basal metabolic rate (kcal/d) calculated by Harris-Benedict equation (presented later in this chapter); V_E = minute ventilation (L/min); T_{max} = maximum daily body temperature (degrees Celsius).

Swinamer Equation

The Swinamer equation is as follows (8):

$$BMR = BSA(945) + A(6.4) + T(108) + RR(24.2) + VT(81.7) - 4349$$

Where: BMR = basal metabolic rate (kcal/d); BSA = body surface area (m^2); T = body temperature degrees Celsius; RR = respiratory rate (breaths/min); VT = tidal volume (L/min).

Ireton-Jones Equation (1992)

The 1992 Ireton-Jones equation for estimated energy expenditure in ventilator-dependent patients is as follows (9):

$$EEE = 1924 - 11(A) + 5(W) + 244(G) + 239(T) + 804(B)$$

Where: EEE = estimated energy expenditure (kcal/d); A = age (years); W = weight (kg); G = gender (female = 0; male = 1); T = diagnosis of trauma (absent = 0; present = 1); B = diagnosis of burn (absent = 0; present = 1).

Harris-Benedict Equation

As noted earlier in this chapter, ADA's Evidence Analysis Library (5) does not recommend the use of the Harris-Benedict equation (HBE) to calculate BEE in critically ill patients. However, HBE is incorporated in the Penn State equation 2003a, and for that reason it is presented here (10):

$$Men: BEE = 66.5 + 13.8(W) + 5.0(H) - 6.8(A)$$

$$Women: BEE = 655.1 + 9.6(W) + 1.9(H) - 4.7(A)$$

Where: BEE = basal energy expenditure (kcal/d); W = weight (kg); H = height (cm); A = age (years).

HYPOCALORIC REGIMEN FOR OBESE PATIENTS
(BMI ≥ 30)

The hypocaloric regimen for obese patients without renal or hepatic dysfunction is **22 kcal/kg ideal body weight** (11,12). (See Chapter 5 for more on ideal body weight.) Both acutely ill and critically ill obese patients have been studied using this caloric approach.

For patients with renal or hepatic dysfunction, the following recommendation from the ADA Evidence Analysis Library (5) may be useful: "If predictive equations are needed for critically ill mechanically ventilated individuals who are obese, consider using Ireton-Jones, 1992, or Penn State, 1998, as they have the best prediction accuracy of equations studied. In some individuals, errors between predicted and actual energy needs will result in under- or over-feeding. *Fair, Conditional.*"

PROTEIN REQUIREMENTS

Protein requirements are based on nutritional status (degree of malnutrition), degree of stress of disease or injury, and physiological capability to metabolize and utilize protein. Nitrogen balance compares nitrogen (protein) intake to nitrogen (protein) output.

For the metabolically stressed patient, current clinical practice dictates providing energy to meet metabolic demand, and, assuming adequate organ function, allows 1.5 g of protein/kg/d. Provision of protein in excess of this amount does not normally improve nitrogen balance, although additional protein may be warranted in certain situations.

A reduction in protein provision may be indicated when hepatic and/or renal dysfunction is present. However, automatic protein restriction in these situations is not appropriate. Nutritional status, clinical condition, and use of renal replacement therapy will affect the protein requirement. Close monitoring of nutritional status is essential if protein intake is restricted (see Table 6.1) (11–15).

Table 6.1 Daily Protein Requirement for Adults

Condition Descriptor	Protein Requirement
DRI reference	0.8 g/kg
Adult maintenance	0.8–1 g/kg
Older adults	1 g/kg
Renal disease: predialysis	0.6–0.8 g/kg
	1.1–1/4 g/kg
Renal disease: hemodialysis, peritoneal dialysis, CRRT	1.2–1.3 g/kg, up to 1.5–1.8 g/kg > 1.5–2.5 g/kg
Hepatitis (acute or chronic)	1–1.5 g/kg
Cirrhosis	1–1.2 g/kg
Encephalopathy, acute	0.6–0.8 g/kg, branched chain amino acids if refractory
Encephalopathy, chronic	0.6–0.8 g/kg, standard protein
Cancer	1–1.5 g/kg
Cancer cachexia	1.5–2.5 g/kg
Bone marrow transplant	1.5 g/kg
Inflammatory bowel disease	1–1.5 g/kg
Short bowel syndrome	1.5–2 g/kg
BMI > 27, normal renal and hepatic function	1.5–2 g/kg/ideal body weight/d (with hypocaloric feeding)
Obesity class I or II, trauma (ICU)	1.9 g/kg ideal body weight/d (with hypocaloric feeding)
Obesity class III, trauma (ICU)	2.5 g/kg/ideal body weight/d (with hypocaloric feeding)
Solid organ transplant: acute posttransplant	1.5–2 g/kg
Solid organ transplant: long-term	1 g/kg
Pregnancy	+ 25 g
Pulmonary disease	1.2–1.5 g/kg
Critical illness (including burns, sepsis, and traumatic brain injury)	1.5–2 g/kg
Stroke	1–1.25 g/kg

Abbreviations: BMI, body mass index; CRRT, continuous renal replacement therapy; DRI, Dietary Reference Intake; ICU, intensive care unit.

Source: Data are from references 11–15.

FLUID MANAGEMENT (16–18)

The goals of fluid management include maintenance of adequate hydration, tissue perfusion, and electrolyte balance. Insensible losses, measured losses (stool, urine, drainage) and alterations in fluid balance due to metabolic changes (fever and hyperthyroidism) or medical therapy (diuretics) must be carefully considered.

No single laboratory test is diagnostic for volume status changes. Clinical examination, along with laboratory monitoring and in some cases hemodynamic monitoring, is needed to appropriately assess and treat fluid and electrolyte abnormalities. In addition, knowledge of the composition of body fluids will enable the clinician to make decisions regarding appropriate replacement strategies for fluid and electrolytes (see Tables 6.2–6.4 and Boxes 6.1–6.5).

Table 6.2   Volume and Electrolyte Composition of Selected Body Fluids

| | Electrolytes (mEq/L) | | | | |
Fluid	Na^+	K^+	Cl^-	HCO_3^-	Volume (L/d)
Saliva	10–30	20–30	10–35	15–30	1–1.5
Gastric, pH < 4	60	10	90		2.5
Gastric, pH > 4	100	10	100		2
Bile	145	5	100–110	35–40	1.5
Duodenal	140	5	80	50	
Pancreatic	140	5	75	90	0.7–1
Ileal	130–140	5–10	104–110	30	3–3.5
Cecal	80	20	50	20	
Colonic	60	30	40	20	0.5–2
Sweat	50	5	55		0–3
New ileostomy	130	20	110	30	0.5–2
Adapted ileostomy	50	5	30	25	0.4
Colostomy	50	10	40	20	0.3–2

Reprinted with permission from Lyerly H, Gaynor J. *The Handbook of Surgical Intensive Care.* 3rd ed. St. Louis, MO: Mosby; 1992:410. Copyright © Mosby 1992.

Table 6.3 Electrolyte Concentrations and Osmolality of Common Intravenous Fluids

Intravenous Fluid	Sodium (mEq/L)	Potassium (mEq/L)	Calcium (mEq/L)	Chloride (mEq/L)	Lactate (mEq/L)	Osmolality (mOsm/L)
5% dextrose solution	0	0	0	0	0	278
10% dextrose solution	0	0	0	0	0	505
0.9% NaCl (normal saline) solution	154	0	0	154	0	308
Sodium lactate solution	167	0	0	0	167	334
5% dextrose, 0.45% NaCl (half normal saline) solution	77	0	0	77	0	406
5% dextrose, 0.9% NaCl (normal saline) solution	154	0	0	154	0	560
Ringer's solution	147.5	4	4.5	156	0	309
Lactated Ringer's solution	130	4	3	109	28	273
5% dextrose in Ringer's solution	147.5	4	4.5	156	0	561
5% dextrose in lactated Ringer's solution	130	4	3	109	28	525

Reprinted with permission from Matarese L, Gottschlich M, eds. *Contemporary Nutrition Support Practice.* 2nd ed. Philadelphia, PA: WB Saunders; 2003:127. Copyright © 2003 WB Saunders.

Table 6.4   Factors That Affect Fluid Requirements

Factor	Increase in Fluid Requirement
Fever	12.5% for each 1°C above normal
Sweating	10%–25%
Hyperventilation	10%–60%
Hyperthyroidism	25%–50%
Extraordinary gastric and/or renal fluid losses	Varies (base adjustment on average 24-hr output)

Reprinted with permission from Matarese L, Gottschlich M, eds. *Contemporary Nutrition Support Practice*. Philadelphia, PA: WB Saunders; 1998:131. Copyright © 1998 WB Saunders.

Box 6.1   Electrolyte Supplementation Guidelines: Magnesium

Comments
- Magnesium sulfate = 8 mEq Mg/g

Enteral Route
- Up to 2 mEq/kg body weight if normal renal function for repletion
- 10 mL milk of magnesia or 600 mg Mg oxide = 20 mEq Mg
- Gastrointestinal tolerance can be a limiting factor

Parenteral Route
- 32–64 mEq magnesium sulfate, up to 1.5 mEq/kg, for severe hypomagnesemia (serum level < 1.0 mg/dL)
- 8–32 mEq magnesium sulfate, up to 1 mEq/kg, for mild to moderate hypomagnesemia (serum level 1.0–1.5 mg/dL)
- May require several days to correct
- Reduce doses by ~50% for persons with renal impairment

Source: Data are from references 15–18.

Box 6.2   Electrolyte Supplementation Guidelines: Phosphorus

Commnents
- 1 mmol = 31 mg elemental phosphorus
- Potassium phosphate preferred over sodium phosphate when serum potassium level < 4.0 mEq/L

Enteral Route
- Sodium phosphate 5 mL three times per day (4.2 mmol phos/mL) or potassium phosphate (1.25 g: 8 mmol phos, 14.2 mEq K) for mild asymptomatic hypophosphatemia

Parenteral Route
- 1 mmol/kg for severe hypophosphatemia (serum level < 1.5 mg/dL)
- 0.64 mmol/kg > 6 h for moderate hypophosphatemia (serum level 1.6–2.2 mg/dL)
- 0.32 mmol/kg > 6 h for mild hypophosphatemia (serum level 2.3–3.0 mg/dL)
- Phosphorus administered at a rate not to exceed 7.5 mmol phosphorus/hr
- Reduce doses by ~50% for persons with renal impairment
- Recheck serum levels periodically

Source: Data are from references 15–18.

Box 6.3   Electrolyte Supplementation Guidelines: Potassium

Commnents
- Review EKG for ventricular arrhythmias
- Correct alkalosis
- Correct concurrent hypomagnesemia
- Continuous cardiac monitoring recommended for infusion rates > 10mEq potassium/h

Enteral Route
- 80–120 mEq/d for repletion
- Each dose: 40 mEq via tube or orally
- Potassium supplements are best administered orally in a moderate dosage over a period of days to weeks to achieve full repletion
- Gastrointestinal tolerance can be a limiting factor

Parenteral Route
- Do not exceed 10 mEq/h via peripheral, 40 mEq/h via central; usual IV infusion rate 10–20 mEq/h
- Suggested repletion schedule:
  - Serum level 2.5–3.4 mg/dL: 20–40 mEq
  - Serum level < 2.5 mg/dL: replace 40–80 mEq in divided doses
  - Reduce doses by ~50% for persons with renal impairment

Source: Data are from references 15–18.

Box 6.4   Electrolyte Supplementation Guidelines: Sodium

Commnents
- Consider check of plasma osmolality and urinary sodium
- Do not correct > 50% of calculated Na deficiency in 1st 24 h; correct 1 mEq/h

Enteral Route
- Hypovolemic hypotonic hyponatremia
- Hypervolemic isotonic hyponatremia
- Isovolemic hypotonic hyponatremia
- Severe symptomatic hyponatremia

Parenteral Route
- Isotonic saline
- Fluid restriction, +/– diuresis
- Fluid restriction
- 3% hypertonic NaCL until Na > 120 mg/dL

Source: Data are from references 15–18.

Box 6.5   Calculation of Fluid Deficit

Body H_2O deficit = Normal – Current TBW
Normal TBW (L) = % TBW × Normal body weight (kg)

$$\text{Current TBW (L)} = \frac{\text{Normal serum Na}^+ \text{ (140 mEq/L)}}{\text{Measured serum Na}^+ \text{ (mEq/L)}} \times$$

Normal TBW (L)

Alternatively, based on algebraic manipulation of the above equations, calculated H_2O deficit

= % TBW × Normal body weight (kg) ×

$$\left[1 - \frac{\text{Normal serum Na}^+ \text{ (140 mEq/L)}}{\text{Measured serum Na}^+ \text{ (mEq/L)}} \right]$$

Reprinted with permission from Matarese L, Gottschlich M, eds. *Contemporary Nutrition Support Practice*. Philadelphia, PA: WB Saunders;1998:131. Copyright © 1998 WB Saunders.

Equations for Estimating Fluid Needs

Holliday-Segar Method (17)

Table 6.5   Calculation of Daily Water Requirements

Body Weight	Water Requirement
< 10 kg	100 mL/kg
11–20 kg	1000 mL + 50 mL/kg for each kg > 10 kg
> 20 kg	1500 mL + 20 mL/kg for each kg > 20 kg

Source: Data are from reference 17.

Body Surface Area Method

1500 mL/m^2

RDA Method

1 mL fluid per 1 kcal of estimated needs

VITAMIN AND MINERAL REQUIREMENTS: DIETARY REFERENCE INTAKES

According to the Institute of Medicine Food and Nutrition Board (19), "the Dietary Reference Intakes (DRIs) are a set of values that serve as standards for nutrient intakes for healthy persons in the United States and Canada." The following points from the Institute of Medicine are important to understanding the DRIs (19):

- The current values were established between 1997 and 2004. They cover 46 nutrient substances.
- DRI values are developed for different sex and age groups (and for pregnant and lactating women). Different groups have different DRI values.

- DRI values are based on average requirements (or average adverse intakes) and provide reliable information on the needs of groups of persons. However, because they are average values, DRIs cannot be used to ensure adequate or safe levels of intake for any single person. DRI values can be used as a guide for individuals but an individual's actual requirement or adverse intake level may be more or less than the DRI value.

The Institute of Medicine has categorized DRIs as follows (20):

- **Adequate Intake (AI)**: The recommended average daily intake level based on observed or experimentally determined approximations or estimates of nutrient intake by a group (or groups) of apparently healthy people that are assumed to be adequate; used when an RDA cannot be determined.
- **Estimated Average Requirement (EAR)**: The average daily nutrient intake level that is estimated to meet the requirements of half the healthy individuals in a particular life stage and gender group.
- **Recommended Dietary Allowance (RDA)**: The average daily dietary nutrient intake level that is sufficient to meet the nutrient requirements of nearly all (97%–98%) healthy individuals in a particular life stage and gender group.
- **Tolerable Upper Intake Level (UL)**: The highest average daily nutrient intake level that is likely to pose no risk of adverse health effects to almost all individuals in the general population. As intake increases above the UL, the potential risk of adverse effects may increase.

- **Acceptable Macronutrient Distribution Ranges (AMDR):** The range of intakes of an energy source that is associated with a reduced risk of chronic disease yet can provide adequate amounts of essential nutrients.

Table 6.6   Dietary Reference Intakes

Component	RDA in bold; AI, not bold	UL
Protein	10%–35% of kcal	
Carbohydrate	45%–65% of kcal	
Fat	20%–35% of kcal	
Fiber (g/d)	Males: < 50 y: 38 > 50 y: 30 Females: < 50 y: 25 > 50 y: 21	
Water/fluid	30 mL/kcal or a minimum of 1500 mL/d	
Arsenic	Not established	ND for all ages
Biotin (µg/d)	> 18 y: 30 Pregnancy: 30 Lactation: 35	Not established
Boron (mg/d)	Not established	20 for all > 18 y
Calcium (mg/d)	19–50 y: 1000 > 50 y: 1200 Pregnancy and lactation do not change requirement	2500 for all > 1 y
Choline (mg/d)	Males > 18 y: 550 Females > 18 y: 425 Pregnancy: < 19 y: 450 > 19 y: 450 Lactation: < 19 y: 550 > 19 y: 550	3500 3500 3000 3500 3000 3500

(continues next page)

Table 6.6 Dietary Reference Intakes (continued)

Component	RDA in bold; AI, not bold	UL

Chromium (µg/d)	Males:
	  14–50 y: 35
	  > 50 y: 30
	Females:
	  19–50 y: 25
	  > 50 y: 20
	Pregnancy:
	  < 19 y: 29
	  > 19 y: 30
	Lactation:
	  < 19 y: 44
	  > 19 y: 45
		ND for all

Copper (µg/d)	> 18 y: **900**
	Pregnancy:
	  < 19: **1000**
	  > 19: **1000**
	Lactation:
	  < 19: **1300**
	  > 19: **1300**
		10,000
		
		8000
		10,000
		
		8000
		10,000

Fluoride (mg/d)	Males > 18 y: **4** Females > 18 y: **3**	10 for all ≥ 9 y

Folate (µg/d), also known as folic acid, folacin, pterolypoly-glutamates
Given as dietary folate equivalents (DFE)
1 DFE = 1 µg food folate = 0.6 µg of folate as a fortified food or as a supplement consumed with food = 0.5 µg of a supplement taken on an empty stomach
	> 18 y: **400**
	Pregnancy:
	  < 19 y: **600**
	  > 19 y: **600**
	Lactation:
	  < 19 y: **500**
	  > 19 y: **500**
		1000
		
		800
		1000
		
		800
		1000

(continues next page)

Table 6.6   Dietary Reference Intakes (continued)

Component	RDA in bold; AI, not bold	UL
Iodine (μg/d)	> 18 y: **150**	1100
	Pregnancy:	
	< 19 y: **220**	900
	> 19 y: **220**	1100
	Lactation:	
	< 19 y: **290**	900
	> 19 y: **290**	1100
Iron (mg/d)	Males > 18 y: **8**	45
	Females:	
	19–50 y: **18**	45
	> 50 y: **8**	45
	Pregnancy: **27**	45
	Lactation:	
	< 19 y: **10**	45
	> 19 y: **9**	45
Magnesium (mg/d)	Males:	350 for all ≥ 9 y
	19–30 y: **400**	
	> 30 y: **420**	
	Females:	
	19–30 y: **310**	
	> 30 y: **320**	
	Pregnancy:	
	< 19 y: **400**	
	19–30 y: **350**	
	> 30 y: **360**	
	Lactation:	
	< 19 y: **360**	
	19–30 y: **310**	
	> 30 y: **320**	
Manganese (mg/d)	Males > 18 y: 2.3	11
	Females > 18 y: 1.8	11
	Pregnancy:	
	< 19 y: 2.0	9
	> 19 y: 2.0	11
	Lactation:	
	< 19 y: 2.6	9
	> 19 y: 2.6	11

(continues next page)

Table 6.6   Dietary Reference Intakes (continued)

Component	RDA in bold; AI, not bold	UL
Molybdenum (μg/d)	> 18 y: **45**	2000
	Pregnancy and lactation: **50**	2000
Niacin (mg/d)	Males > 18 y: **16**	35
Given as niacin	Females > 18 y: **14**	35
equivalents (NE).	Pregnancy:	
1 mg of niacin = 60	< 19 y: **18**	30
mg of tryptophan;	> 19 y: **18**	35
0–6 mo = preformed	Lactation:	
niacin (not NE)	< 19 y: **17**	30
	> 19 y: **17**	35
Nickel (mg/d)	Not established	1.0 for all > 13 y
Pantothenic Acid (mg/d)	> 14 y: 5	ND for all ages
	Pregnancy: 6	
	Lactation: 7	
Phosphorus (mg/d)	> 18 y: **700**	4000 for > 18–70
		3000 for > 70
	Pregnancy:	
	< 19 y: **1250**	3500
	> 19 y: **700**	3500
	Lactation:	
	< 19 y: **1250**	4000
	> 19 y: **700**	4000
Riboflavin (mg/d),	Males > 13 y: **1.3**	Not established
also known as	Females: > 18 y: **1.1**	
Vitamin B-2	Pregnancy: **1.4**	
	Lactation: **1.6**	
Selenium (μg/d)	> 13 y: **55**	400
	Pregnancy: **60**	400
	Lactation: **70**	400
Silicon	Not established	ND
Thiamin (mg/d), also	Males > 13 y: **1.2**	Not established
known as Vitamin	Females: > 18 y: **1.1**	
B-1 or aneurin	Pregnancy: **1.4**	
	Lactation: **1.4**	

(continues next page)

Table 6.6   Dietary Reference Intakes (continued)

Component	RDA in bold; AI, not bold	UL
Vanadium (mg/d)	Not established	Females who are pregnant or lactating: ND Males and females > 18 (nonpregnant, nonlactating): 1.8
Vitamin A (µg/d) Includes provitamin A carotenoids that are dietary precursors of retinol Values are given as retinol activity equivalents (RAEs). 1 RAE = 12 µg retinol, 12 µg ß carotene, 24 µg a carotene, or 24 µg ß cryptoxanthin. Divide retinol equivalents (REs) from provitamin A carotenoids in foods by 2 to determine RAEs. For preformed vitamin A carotenoids in supplements, 1 RE = 1 RAE.	Males > 18 y: **900** Females > 18 y: **700** Pregnancy: < 19 y: **750** > 19 y: **770** Lactation: < 19 y: **1200** > 19 y: **1300**	3000 2800 3000 2800 3000 2800
Vitamin B-6 (mg/d) Comprises a group of six related compounds: pyridoxal, pyridoxine, pyridoxamine, and 5'-phosphates (pyridoxal phosphate, pyridoxine phosphate, pyridoxamine phosphate)	Males: 19–50 y: **1.3** > 50 y: **1.7** Females: 19–50 y: **1.3** > 50 y: **1.5** Pregnancy: < 19 y: **1.9** > 19 y: **1.9** Lactation: < 19 y: **2.0** > 19 y: **2.0**	100 100 80 100 80 100 80 100

(continues next page)

Table 6.6 Dietary Reference Intakes (continued)

Component	RDA in bold; AI, not bold	UL

Vitamin B-12 (µg/d), also known as cobalamin	> 18 y: **2.4**
	Pregnancy:
	  < 19 y: **2.6**
	  > 19 y: **2.6**
	Lactation:
	  < 19 y: **2.8**
	  > 19 y: **2.8**
		Not established

Vitamin C (mg/d), also known as ascorbic acid, dehydroxoascorbic acid (DHA)	Males:
	  > 18 y: **90**
	Females:
	  > 18 y: **75**
	Pregnancy:
	  < 19 y: **80**
	  > 19 y: **85**
	Lactation:
	  < 19 y: **115**
	  > 19 y: **120**
		2000
		
		2000
		
		1800
		2000
		
		1800
		2000

Vitamin D (µg/d), also known as calciferol 1 µg calciferol = 40 IU vitamin D DRI values are based on the absence of adequate exposure to sunlight	Birth to 50 y: 5 51–70 y: 10 > 70 y: 15 Pregnancy and lactation: 5	50 for all > 1 y

Vitamin E (mg/d), also known as alpha-tocopherol	Males:
	  > 18 y: **15**
	Females:
	  > 18 y: **15**
	Pregnancy:
	  < 19 y: **15**
	  > 19 y: **15**
	Lactation:
	  < 19 y: **19**
	  > 19 y: **19**
		1000
		
		1000
		
		800
		1000
		
		800
		1000

(continues next page)

Table 6.6   Dietary Reference Intakes (continued)

Component	RDA in bold; AI, not bold	UL
Vitamin K (µg/d)	Males > 18 y: 120	ND for all ages
	Females > 18 y: 90	
	Pregnancy:	
	< 19 y: 75	
	> 19 y: 90	
	Lactation:	
	< 19 y: 75	
	> 19 y: 90	
Zinc (mg/d)	Males > 19 y: **11**	40
	Females > 18 y: **8**	40
	Pregnancy:	
	< 19 y: **12**	34
	> 19 y: **11**	40
	Lactation:	
	< 19 y: **13**	34
	> 19 y: **12**	40

Abbreviation: ND = not determinable because of lack of data on adverse effects in age group and because of concern about inability to handle excess amounts. Sources of intake should be from food only, to prevent high levels of intake.

Source: Reference 21: Institute of Medicine. Dietary Reference Intakes (DRIs) Summary Table. http://www.iom.edu/CMS/3788/4574/45132/45134.aspx. Accessed December 29, 2007.

REFERENCES

1. American Dietetic Association Evidence Analysis Library. Determination of Resting Metabolic Rate. http://www.ada evidencelibrary.com/topic.cfm?cat=2954. Accessed November 3, 2007.

2. American Dietetic Association Evidence Analysis Library. Adult Weight Management (AWM) Determination of Resting Metabolic Rate. http://www.adaevidencelibrary.com/template .cfm?template=guide_summary&key=621. Accessed November 3, 2007.

3. Mifflin MD, St. Jeor ST, Hill LA, Scott BJ, Daugherty SA, Koh YO. A new predictive equation for resting energy expenditure in healthy individuals. *Am J Clin Nutr.* 1990;51:241–247.

4. Ireton-Jones CS, Jones JD. Should predictive equations or indirect calorimetry be used to design nutrition support regimens? Predictive equations should be used. *Nutr Clin Pract.* 1998;13:141–143.

5. American Dietetic Association Evidence Analysis Library. Critical Illness (CI) Determination of Resting Metabolic Rate (RMR). http://www.adaevidencelibrary.com/template.cfm?key=1309. Accessed November 3, 2007.

6. American Dietetic Association Evidence Analysis Library. Critical Illness (CI) Respiratory Quotient as a Method to Detect Measurement Error. http://www.adaevidencelibrary.com/template.cfm?key=1006&auth=1. Accessed November 3, 2007.

7. Frankenfield D, Smith JS, Cooney RN. Validation of 2 approaches to predicting resting metabolic rate in critically ill patients. *JPEN J Parenter Enteral Nutr.* 2004;28:259–264.

8. Swinamer DL, Grace MG, Hamilton SM, Jones RL, Roberts P, King EG. Predictive equation for assessing energy expenditure in mechanically ventilated critically ill patients. *Crit Care Med.* 1990;18:657–661.

9. Ireton Jones CS, Turner WW, Leipa GU, Baxter CR. Equations for the estimation of energy expenditure for patients with burns with special reference to ventilatory status. *J Burn Care Rehabil.* 1992;13:330–333.

10. Harris JA, Benedict FG. *Biometric Studies of Basal Metabolism in Man.* Washington, DC: Carnegie Institution of Washington; 1919. Publication no. 270.

11. Choban PS, Burge JC, Scales D, Flancbaum L. Hypoenergetic nutrition support in hospitalized obese patients: a simplified method for clinical application. *Am J Clin Nutr.* 1997;66:546–550.

12. Dickerson RN. Hypocaloric feeding of obese patients in the intensive care unit. *Curr Opin Clin Nutr Metab Care.* 2005;8:189–196.

13. Mahan K, Escott-Stump S, eds. *Krause's Food, Nutrition, and Diet Therapy.* 12th ed. Philadelphia, PA: WB Saunders; 2008.

14. Matarese L, Gottschlich M, eds. *Contemporary Nutrition Support Practice.* 2nd ed. Philadelphia, PA: WB Saunders; 2003.

15. Gottschlich MM, ed. *The A.S.P.E.N. Nutrition Support Core Curriculum. A Case-Based Approach—the Adult Patient.* Silver Spring, MD: American Society for Parenteral and Enteral Nutrition; 2007.

16. Whitmire S. Fluids and electrolytes. In: Matarese L, Gottschlich M, eds. *Contemporary Nutrition Support Practice*. Philadelphia, PA: WB Saunders; 2003:122–144.

17. Lyerly H, Gaynor J. *The Handbook of Surgical Intensive Care.* 3rd ed. St. Louis, MO: Mosby; 1992.

18. Brown KA, Dickerson RN, Morgan LM, Alexander KH, Minard G, Brown RO. A new graduated dosing regimen for phosphorus replacement in patients receiving nutrition support. *JPEN J Parenter Enteral Nutr.* 2006;30:209–214.

19. Institute of Medicine. Dietary Reference Intakes. http://www.iom.edu/CMS/3788/4574.aspx. Accessed December 29, 2007.

20. Institute of Medicine. DRI Values: Definitions. http://www.iom.edu/CMS/3788/4574/45105.aspx. Accessed December 29, 2007.

21. Institute of Medicine. Dietary Reference Intakes (DRIs) Summary Table. http://www.iom.edu/CMS/3788/4574/45132/45134.aspx. Accessed December 29, 2007.

chapter 7

The Nutrition Care Process

PAMELA CHARNEY, PhD, RD

The House of Delegates of the American Dietetic Association (ADA) approved the Nutrition Care Process and Model (NCPM) in order to meet professional goals as established by ADA's Strategic Plan (1). These goals include:

- Increasing demand and utilization of services provided by members and
- Empowering members to compete successfully in a rapidly changing environment.

WHAT IS THE NUTRITION CARE PROCESS AND MODEL?

The NCPM is a standardized process that promotes individualized care and is *not* simply a method to provide standardized care (2). The NCPM is defined as "a systematic problem-solving method that dietetics professionals use to critically think and make decisions to address nutrition-related problems and provide safe and effective quality nutrition care" (2). The purpose of the NCPM is to give dietetics professionals a "consistent and systematic structure and method by which to think critically and make decisions" (2).

The visual representation of the NCPM includes two outer rings describing external and internal factors that affect the dietetics practice of the registered dietitian (RD) (2). These factors are listed in Table 7.1.

Table 7.1   External and Internal Factors That Affect Dietetics Practice

Type of Factor	Examples
External	• Health care systems • Financing • Socioeconomic factors • Regulatory agencies
Intrinsic	• Code of ethics • Standards of practice • Standards of professional performance • Dietetics knowledge and experience • Collaborative networks

In the NCPM graphic (2), the two outer rings surround the four steps of the Nutrition Care Process, represented by four quadrants at the center of the model:

- Nutrition Assessment
- Nutrition Diagnosis
- Nutrition Intervention
- Nutrition Monitoring and Evaluation

Although the steps build on each other, the process supports reassessment and/or modification of care at each step.

Box 7.1 defines each step in the Nutrition Care Process and provides supporting key concepts of each step. Additional detailed information regarding the NCP is also available from ADA (http://www.eatright.org).

Box 7.1   The Steps of the Nutrition Care Process

Step 1: Nutrition Assessment
Obtain adequate information to identify nutrition-related problems.
Nutrition assessment is initiated by a referral and/or screening
process. Nutrition assessment is a systematic process of obtaining,
verifying, and interpreting data in order to make decisions about the
nature and cause of nutrition-related problems.

Key supporting components:[a]
• Food and nutrition history
• Biochemical data, medical tests, and procedures
• Anthropometric measurements
• Physical examination findings
• Client history

Step 2: Nutrition Diagnosis
The identification and labeling that describes a nutrition problem that
dietetics professionals are responsible for treating independently.

Key supporting components:
• **Nutrition diagnosis**: Alterations in the client's nutritional status
  are described in the nutrition diagnostic statement.
• **Etiology**: The cause or etiology of the nutrition problem. For
  example, involuntary weight loss may be related to continued
  malabsorption due to radiation enteritis.
• **Signs and symptoms**: Signs are the findings of the health care
  professional (eg, temperature, pulse, weight, body mass index).
  Symptoms are the reasons that a patient or client seeks health care.

The nutrition diagnostic statement should be written in a PES format
that states the Problem (P), Etiology (E), and Signs and Symptoms (S).

Step 3: Nutrition Intervention
A specific set of activities and associated materials used to address
the problem. The nutrition intervention includes planning, and
implementing the appropriate interventions/activities that facilitate to
change a nutrition-related behavior, risk factor, or to meet the client's
nutrition needs.

Key supporting components:
• The nutrition intervention plan prioritizes the nutrition diagnoses
  based on severity of the problem, client's needs and goals, and
  benefits/risks.
• Patient-focused clinical outcomes are identified for each nutrition
  diagnosis.

(continues next page)

Box 7.1   The Steps of the Nutrition Care Process (continued)

- Relevant, accurate, and timely documentation supports the goals of the planned nutrition interventions, including specific goals and expected outcomes.
- Documentation should also include adjustments in plan, client/caregiver's perception and compliance, plan for follow-up, and resources needed.
- Evidence-based practice and intervention guidelines, current research, and outcome management theories, training, and studies.

Step 4. Nutrition Monitoring and Evaluation
Monitoring specifically refers to the review and measurement of the client's status at scheduled follow-up points, pertaining to the nutrition diagnosis, intervention plans/goals, and outcomes. Evaluation is the systematic comparison of current findings with previous status, intervention goals, or a reference standard.

Key supporting components:
- The purpose of monitoring and evaluating is to assess to what degree progress is being made and whether goals/outcomes are being achieved. Selected outcome measures are identified that are related to the client's nutrition needs, nutrition diagnosis, desired goals/outcomes, and clinical status.
- The selected outcome measures should be relevant to the nutrition diagnosis, nutrition goals, the client's clinical status, and quality of life/management goals.
- Reevaluation should compare current status to prior status and outcome goals.
- The monitoring and evaluation process also requires quality documentation that documents progress toward goals, compliance, factors supporting or hindering progress, and nutrition care future plans.

ᵃThese components of Nutrition Assessment are described in detail in each chapter of this pocket guide.

Adapted with permission from Lacey K, Pritchett E. Nutrition care process and model: ADA adopts road map to quality care and outcomes management. *J Am Diet Assoc*. 2003;103:1061–1072.

DIETETICS TERMINOLOGY

A standardized terminology contains an agreed upon set of terms and definitions. Health care professionals have used standardized terminologies for a variety of purposes, including documenting medical diagnosis and services provided. Examples of health care terminologies are listed in Table 7.2.

Table 7.2   Examples of Health Care Terminologies

Terminologies	*Use*
International Classification of Disease (ICD)	To document medical diagnoses for billing purposes
Current Procedural Terminology (CPT)	To bill for services provided
North American Nursing Diagnosis Association (NANDA)	To document nursing diagnosis

NUTRITION DIAGNOSIS

While RDs might be comfortable with nutrition assessment, intervention, and monitoring/evaluation, the concept of identifying a nutrition diagnosis may be unfamiliar. Other health care professions, including medicine, nursing, occupational therapy, and physical therapy, have defined roles as diagnosticians in their domain of practice. The NCP provides a framework for the RD to learn and apply a diagnostic process and thus support a role for the RD as an integral member of the health care team.

How Health Care Professionals Identify a Diagnosis

The NCP focuses on the ability of the RD to use critical thinking and decision-making skills to identify a nutrition diagnosis. Research shows that health care professionals use different strategies in the diagnostic process (3–5). Table 7.3 describes some of those strategies (6,7).

Table 7.3   Diagnostic Reasoning Strategies

Strategy	Description
Hypothetico-deductive reasoning	• Formulation of a set of plausible diagnoses based on early bits of information • Diagnoses ruled in or out based on continual gathering of information • Used by all clinicians; experts are faster and have less information than novices
Pattern recognition	• Used most successfully by experts • Recognize new problems in context of past experience with same patterns • Signs and symptoms conform to previously learned set of signs and symptoms • Must have extensive experience
Scheme-inductive	• Development of framework/road map to create major divisions (chunks) of information • "Diagnostic tree" with branches representing decision points • Similar to algorithmic approach • Used by experts and novices with good success

Source: Data are from references 6 and 7.

PES Statements

RDs have not traditionally been trained to systematically diagnose nutrition problems. The NCP addresses this issue by using the Problem (P), Etiology (E), Signs/Symptoms (S) statement to describe the nutrition diagnosis identified. The *problem* is the nutrition diagnosis—eg, "inadequate oral food/beverage intake" (8). The *etiology* describes the factors associated with development or cause of the problem—eg, "inadequate oral food/beverage intake *related to nausea following antibiotic administration before meals.*" The RD should ensure that the etiology is the direct cause of the nutrition diagnosis and should verify that the nutrition intervention selected can address the etiology. In the case of the etiology described in this paragraph, the RD might collaborate with the clinical pharmacist to alter medication schedules if possible. The *signs and symptoms* are the clinical and subjective findings that the RD used to identify the nutrition problem—eg, "inadequate oral food/beverage intake related to nausea following antibiotic administration *as evidenced by documented intake less than 50% of estimated requirements for past 3 days.*"

Case Study

A 78-year-old woman was admitted to an acute-care facility from a long-term-care (LTC) facility with a presumed diagnosis of pneumonia. She had been doing well until approximately 3 weeks before admission, when symptoms of cough and congestion began. Her symptoms worsened, and she was noted 24 hours ago to be short of breath with a fever of 100° F and a productive cough. During the admission screening process, the patient mentioned to the nurse that she was surprised to note that she'd lost 10 lb during this illness. The nurse consulted the RD for nutrition assessment.

The RD conducted a nutrition assessment and noted the weight loss. Physical exam done by the RD was unremarkable. Biochemical data revealed normal electrolytes, serum glucose 120 g/dL, and albumin 3.4 g/dL. Her medications before admission included a diuretic for mild hypertension. A broad-spectrum antibiotic was ordered on admission to treat the presumed pneumonia. The patient had been residing in the LTC facility for the past 8 months. She has been doing well, and eating most meals, according to the facility RD who also notes that the patient's intake has been slowly decreasing during this illness; the patient had consumed less than half of her meals for the past 3 days. The patient mentioned to the RD that she has had significant nausea associated with coughing spells. She says the nausea seems to "destroy my appetite for meals."

Based on this information, the RD determines that the patient has the following nutrition diagnoses:

- Involuntary weight loss related to coughing spells at meals, as evidenced by a 10-lb weight loss before admission (PES statement).
- Inadequate oral food/beverage intake related to nausea, as evidenced by intake less than 50% of requirement for 3 days.

Once the nutrition diagnoses are identified, the RD must implement nutrition interventions that will best treat the nutrition diagnosis. In this case, the RD could intervene by providing smaller meals, snacks, or other alterations to meals and would monitor the patient's reports of nausea and (given adequate time to see weight change) by monitoring weight. Once discharged, the LTC RD can be asked to continue monitoring the patient's weight.

REFERENCES

1. American Dietetic Association. Mission and vision. http://www.eatright.org. Accessed November 1, 2007.
2. Lacey K, Pritchett E. Nutrition care process and model: ADA adopts road map to quality care and outcomes management. *J Am Diet Assoc.* 2003;103:1061–1072.

3. Botti M. Role of knowledge and ability in student nurses' clinical decision-making. *Nurs Health Sci.* 2003;5:39–49.

4. Cahan A, Gilon D, Manor O, Paltiel O. Probabilistic reasoning and clinical decision-making: do doctors overestimate diagnostic probabilities? *QJM.* 2003;96:763–769.

5. Elstein AS, Schwarz A. Evidence base of clinical diagnosis: clinical problem solving and diagnostic decision making: selective review of the cognitive literature. *BMJ.* 2002;324:729–732.

6. Coderre S, Mandin H, Harasym PH, Fick GH. Diagnostic reasoning strategies and diagnostic success. *Med Educ.* 2003;37:695–703.

7. Sackett DI, Haynes RB, Guyatt GH, Tugwell P. Clinical diagnostic strategies. In: Sackett DI, Haynes RB, Guyatt G, Tugwell P, eds. *Clinical Epidemiology: A Basic Science for Clinical Medicine.* 2nd ed. Philadelphia, PA: Lippincott, Williams & Wilkins; 1991.

8. American Dietetic Association. *International Dietetics and Nutrition Terminology (IDNT) Reference Manual: Standardized Language for the Nutrition Care Process.* Chicago, IL: American Dietetic Association; 2007.

glossary

Alopecia: loss of hair, baldness.

Anasarca: generalized massive edema.

Angular stomatitis: sores or inflammation at corners of the mouth.

Ascites: accumulation of serous fluid in the abdominal cavity.

Ataxia: poor muscular coordination.

Atrophic lingual papillae: slick tongue.

Auscultation: listening for sounds within the body.

Bitot's spot: superficial, triangular, foamy gray spots on conjunctiva of eye, consisting of keratinized epithelium.

Borborygmi: Audible abdominal sound produced by hyperactive intestinal peristalsis.

Cachexia: profound state of muscle and fat wasting.

Cheilosis: dry, cracking, ulcerated lips.

Cheyne-Stokes breathing: Periods of deep breathing alternating with periods of apnea. Can be caused by drug-induced respiratory depression or brain damage.

Chvostek's sign: Twitching of facial muscles due to neuromuscular excitability secondary to hypocalcemia.

Crackles: discontinuous breath sounds. Fine crackles are "popping" noises. Course crackles are lower pitched and more noticeable on expiration.

Diaphoresis: profuse perspiration.

Dullness: diminished resonance with percussion over solid organs.

Ecchymosis: small hemorrhagic spot, which is a nonelevated, rounded, or irregular blue or purplish patch in the skin or mucous membranes. Larger than a petechia.

Flag sign: transverse depigmentation of hair.

Flatness: soft, high-pitched sounds of short duration heard with percussion over structures with no air, such as fat and muscle.

Follicular hyperkeratosis: "goose bumps" that do not go away with warming or rubbing.

Gag reflex: involuntary reflex that protects airway. Test for gag reflex by stimulating the back of the throat lightly on left and right sides.

Glossitis: magenta or scarlet, raw tongue.

Guarding: voluntary tightening of muscles to protect against discomfort/pain.

Heart murmur: swishing or blowing sound resulting from altered blood flow in the heart.

Hypogeusia: decreased sense of taste.

Hyposmia: decreased sense of smell.

Inspection: close examination.

Jaundice: yellow (bile pigment) discoloration of skin, mucous membranes, and sclera as a result of elevated serum bilirubin (also called icterus).

Koilonychia: dystrophy of the fingernails resulting in thin, concave nails with the edges raised. Also called "spoon nail" and is associated with iron deficiency.

Kussmaul breathing: a rapid, deep, and labored breathing, often seen in patients with diabetic ketoacidosis, uremia, or pneumonia. It is also described as "air hunger."

Oliguria: reduced urine output in relation to fluid intake.

Ophthalmoplegia: paralysis of ocular muscles.

Palpation: using the hands, fingertips, and finger pads to apply light to deep pressure to the skin to determine structures beneath the surface and to detect abnormalities.

Paresthesias: numbness and tingling sensation.

Percussion: using short, sharp blows by the fingertips and finger pads to create vibrations in the abdomen, which, in turn, produce sounds that are described according to pitch, duration, and intensity.

Pericardial friction rub: squeaky or rubbing heart sound, caused by inflamed layers of the pericardium rubbing against each other.

Petechia: pinpoint, nonelevated, round, purplish-red spot, which occurs with intradermal or submucosal hemorrhage.

Pitting edema: fluid accumulation in the peripheral tissues, which results in sustained indentation when pressure is applied (1+ = 2 mm, 2+ = 4 mm, 3+ = 6 mm, 4+ = 8 mm).

Pleural friction rub: lung sounds that vary from a few intermittent sounds similar to crackles to harsh grating, creaking, or leathery sounds that occur with respiration.

Purpura: bruising/bleeding into the skin.

Resonance: a loud, low-pitched sound with long duration heard with percussion over the lungs.

Rhonchus: a snoring sound.

Rickets: beading of ribs, epiphyseal swelling, bowlegs.

Seborrhea: scaling of skin around nostrils.

SIADH: syndrome of inappropriate, antidiuretic hormone secretion, characterized by hypertonic urine output, normal GFR, normal or expanded (no edema) total body water, urinary sodium wasting, hypo-osmolality, hyponatremia, and increased ADH release.

Trousseau's sign: muscular contractions of the wrist, fingers, and thumb due to neuromuscular excitability secondary to hypocalcemia.

Tympany: the sound created when percussion is performed over air-filled cavity. Drum or bell-like sound.

Xerosis: abnormal dryness of the eyes.

index

Page number followed by *b* indicates box; *f*, figure; *t*, table.